PERMANENT FAT LOSS
IN 5 SIMPLE STEPS

Body Blitz

JOANNA HALL MSc

Thorsons

Thorsons
An Imprint of HarperCollins*Publishers*
77–85 Fulham Palace Road,
Hammersmith, London W6 8JB

The Thorsons website address is: www.thorsons.com

First published 2001
10 9 8 7 6 5 4 3 2 1

Joanna Hall's website address is: www.activeaction.com

A catalogue record of this book is
available from the British Library

ISBN 0 7225 4043 4

Typeset by Davidson Pre-Press, Glasgow
Printed and bound in Great Britain by
Martins the Printers Ltd, Berwick upon Tweed

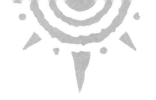

Contents

Acknowledgements

I would like to say a huge thank you to my clients who have been, and are, a joy to work with and whose results with the *Body Blitz* programme have been a constant source of inspiration both to myself and others. Their support through the development of my work has made me feel very privileged.

Thanks to my literary agent Michael Alcock, Wanda Whitely and her great team at HarperCollins, especially Jo Kyle and Sam Grant, and my technical editor and friend Tony Lycholat, who have been brilliant with all their help on *Body Blitz* – my first book publication.

To my colleagues at Activeaction.com I extend a special thanks, especially to Sue and Renee who have been there for advice, support and personal friendship.

PART I: ALL ABOUT BODY BLITZ

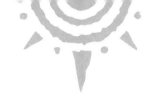

CHAPTER ONE

Be The Best You Can Be!

Most people know to lose weight we have to eat less and exercise more – but somehow something always seems to get in the way – LIFE! Here are a few questions for you to think about:

1. Do you experience frustration at seeing your weight go up and down on the scales?

    a. yes
    b. no

2. Are you a seasoned dieter who tries every diet available and yet you still don't seem able to shift those extra pounds?

    a. yes
    b. no

3. Do your diet attempts leave you a diet hermit rather than living life to the full?

    a. yes
    b. no

4. Do you want a diet and fitness plan that fits in with your lifestyle – that lets you go out to dinner and socialize with friends, while still achieving your weight and fat loss goals?

a. yes

b. no

If you have answered yes to any of the above questions then Body Blitz is for you. The Body Blitz diet and fitness plan shows you the five steps you need take to lose weight and body fat – and keep it off for good!

WHAT IS THE BODY BLITZ PLAN?

Losing weight and body fat is a subject that provokes an array of discussions and fad slimming products and diets. Unfortunately, while some people may claim spectacular results with tablets, potions and 'miracle' foods, the real truth is that long-term weight management requires a little effort and know-how to be able to make it work for you not just for today, but for the future too.

The two keys to successful weight and body fat loss are simple – good nutrition and regular exercise. The challenge comes when we try to fit a healthy diet and exercise into our busy lives – maybe you're running around after your kids all day, or working long hours, or simply leading a jam-packed social life and it feels as though you don't even have time to think about eating well and exercising – let alone do it! This is where Body Blitz steps in. Body Blitz will help you design a diet and fitness plan that fits in with *your* life – just the way it is. This way you can make your own realistic goals, you don't have to make any radical changes to your lifestyle and most importantly, you will achieve your weight and fat loss goals. Body Blitz is about **being the best you can be whilst still living the life you wish to live.**

HOW DOES BODY BLITZ WORK?

Body Blitz contains five steps to help you achieve your weight and body fat goals. The nutritional and exercise strategies contained in these steps have been tried and tested by my weight management clients over the last six years – they have worked for them and they will work for you. Each strategy plays a different role in helping you lose weight and body fat in different lifestyle situations. The five steps are:

1. USE THE STARCH CURFEW

By not eating certain carbohydrates after five p.m. you will lose weight and boost your energy levels. It is a strategy that allows you to cut your overall calorie intake and get the right balance of nutrients at the right time of the day. By eating starch with protein at lunchtime instead of in your evening meal, you will beat your mid-afternoon sugar cravings (the dieter's downfall!) and fuel yourself with energy and brainpower for the rest of the day.

2. DRINK MORE WATER

If you drink less than eight glasses of water a day you may well be chronically dehydrated – this means you will lack energy and your brain will misinterpret this tiredness as a need to eat more food. So by drinking a minimun of two litres of water a day you will fuel yourself with energy, curb your hunger and enhance your nutrient absorption. Stick to the action points in Step Two and you'll be well on the way to a super-hydrated and less hungry body!

3. DECREASE YOUR FAT INTAKE

This is not about cutting all fat from your diet – some fat is essential for our health – instead it is about reducing your overall fat intake whilst at the same time increasing the good sources of fat in your diet. By eating 40 grams of the right fats a day you will soon see your own body fat decrease.

4. BE CONSISTENT

The good news is the best way to lose weight is not to deprive yourself of everything you love, but instead to stick to **the 80–20 rule**. This means rather than being good 100% of the time, if you can stick to the Body Blitz Plan for just 80% of the time you will succeed! Being consistent means you can actually eat a little more and you will still lose weight and body fat and you are not setting yourself up for guilt and 'failure!'

5. MAKE TIME FOR EXERCISE

Most of us know we have to take regular exercise to lose weight. The challenge comes when we try to fit physical activity into our busy lives – Step Five will show you how. The Body Blitz exercise and activity strategies are:

- STRUCTURED EXERCISE SESSIONS

  This is your designated exercise session when you will either be exercising at home, in a gym or outside. These sessions typically last a minimum of 30–60 minutes and you should have three sessions every week.

- ACCUMULATED PHYSICAL ACTIVITY

  This is the energy we burn through moving our bodies physically during our day. You should accumulate 15 minutes physical activity every day.

  It is the combination of your structured exercise sessions and accumulated physical activity that will help you feel healthier and more energetic and help you to achieve your weight and body fat goals.

You will also find in Body Blitz over 25 recipes for healthy eating and to help you put the starch curfew into practice, as well as a 14-day eating plan. Everything in this book has been tested by real people with real pressures and their own stories and tips will help you be in control against unwanted excess weight and body fat.

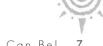

IT'S NEVER TOO LATE TO START!

LET'S MEET FRED

Fred was the high school sporting hero – he was on every sports team and he loved being mauled on the rugby pitch; he was fit and active and he naturally attracted attention. Fifteen years on things are a little different. Fred expends his energy sitting behind a desk and attending business lunches. He gets out of breath walking up a hill and his shirt collars and trousers are feeling a little tight. He reads about the risk of heart disease and obesity but – well, he was the sporting hero at school, he was fit! These things don't affect people like him – or so he thinks.

NOW LET'S MEET MARY

Mary hated sport at school. She was the bookworm who could not understand how others could be happy to get cold and wet on a hockey field in the middle of the cold, grey winter. She much preferred to sneak off somewhere and have a donut and hot chocolate. Fifteen years on things are a little different – she still hates the thought of getting cold and wet for the sake of sport, and she still enjoys the occasional donut, but she has started getting active! She walks whenever she can – even though it is not always as much as she would like to because she's got three children and an elderly relative to look after. But she expends a lot of energy in her daily chores and she always takes the stairs and never the lift! Mary feels better! She no longer finds herself out of breath when she walks up a hill. She looks trim and healthy.

It's never too late to start being active – in fact, being active in your later years can be even more important than being active in your younger days. Long-term studies suggest that being active with sport at school has NO protective effect against heart disease, breast cancer and weight gain if you do not remain active in your adult life. Becoming active now and staying active has an immediate protective effect on your health! It's never too late to start!

LIVE THE LIFE YOU WISH TO LIVE!

Have you ever beaten yourself up for breaking your new diet that promises to shrink you into your favourite jeans that you could fit into five years ago, within seven days? Or forgotten to go to the gym for a week and on the eighth day, the time you would normally be in the gym, you find yourself propping up the bar with a bowl of bar snacks and a bottle of wine? If you can relate to either of these scenarios then the Body Blitz diet and fitness plan is definitely for you. Body Blitz shows you that the key to long-term successful weight management is not to deprive yourself of everything you love or to beat yourself up when you fail – it is about developing and appreciating a balanced and consistent approach to eating and exercise, where you only have to be 'good' 80% of the time and you will succeed.

In short, Body Blitz is about helping you develop strategies that allow you to enjoy the things you want to enjoy, whilst incorporating some healthy activities at the same time to help you realize your weight and body fat goals. By following the five steps in the Body Blitz Plan, you will have the confidence and know-how to say goodbye to excess weight and body fat – for good!

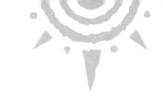

CHAPTER TWO

The Body Blitz Lifestyle

Today's lifestyle throws temptation at us 24 hours a day, 7 days a week and 365 days a year. Supermarkets re-circulate the smells of their bakery ovens back into the store, ready-prepared foods are becoming more and more convenient and fast food ever more accessible with tempting fare brought right to our front door!

The world we live in today is perpetually stimulating our minds and taste buds to eat more than we need – to the point where we are almost living in a food-toxic environment. At the same time our society enables us to become less and less active. We are under pressure to achieve more things in one day but the irony is with the wonders of modern technology this results in us expending less physical energy.

Everybody knows that a healthy lifestyle makes sense – not just for today but also for our future health and wellbeing. But somehow our good intentions never seem to have much staying power. Perhaps it is the thought of a life with-out a curry or the thought of an existence of carrot sticks and lettuce leaves, but the whole process can seem very unappealing. Then there is the interminable pounding of our bodies in the gym – only to have burnt off the equivalent of a mini Mars bar! All in all, it is enough to make you reach for the pizza home delivery number and the TV remote control!

But living a healthy life does not mean you have to live a life without choco-late or alcohol. The Body Blitz Plan is about being the best you can be whilst living the life you wish to live. It is about making small changes matter. It is about enjoying life while putting the Body Blitz strategies into place and knowing how to make lifestyle decisions work for you. In short, it is about applying a bit of know-how so that you can have your cake and eat it and pick your dress and wear it!

GETTING YOUR DIET RIGHT

The first thing we need to look at with the Body Blitz Plan is our diet. It is very important to get the fundamentals of our diet right with the right nutrients in the right balance. A good diet includes food from each of the four nutrient food groups. These food groups are:

- Carbohydrates
- Proteins
- Fats
- Water

CARBOHYDRATES

Carbohydrates form the backbone of our diet. Fruit, vegetables, simple sugars such as biscuits and cakes, and starches such as potatoes, rice and bread are all carbohydrates. Carbohydrate-rich foods supply the body with its primary source of fuel – glucose. Glucose is a type of sugar which the body can easily use and transport – when we talk about blood sugars we are actually talking about our blood glucose levels. Glucose can be stored in the muscles as glycogen and is the main source of fuel for our working muscles, the nervous system and brain. We will be talking more about carbohydrates and starch in Step One.

PROTEINS

Proteins are essential for tissue repair, maintenance and growth. They are crucial for our health as they make up part of every cell in the body. A regular supply of protein is required in the diet to compensate for the continual loss that occurs in the body. Proteins are made up of smaller units called amino acids. Not all proteins contain all the essential amino acids required by our bodies – this is why if we are vegetarian we need to ensure that we have a variety of protein sources to ensure our bodies are getting a complete range of the necessary proteins. Protein can be divided into two groups: dairy products, which include cheese, yoghurt, eggs and non-dairy sources, which include meat, fish, pulses and beans. The important role that protein plays in repairing the body means that it is much harder for the body to store excess protein as body fat in the cells.

DIETARY FATS

Dietary fats come from a variety of sources. There are various ways of defining fats but one of the simplest is to consider fats as visible and invisible. Visible fats are, as the name suggests, foods that we can see are made of fat. Cheese, butter, oils and creams are examples of visible fats. Invisible fats are foods with a predominant fat content although we may not be aware of it: examples include coconut, avocado and egg yolks. Fats are divided into three groups: saturated, polyunsaturated and monounsaturated. Saturated fats (including trans fats) are non-essential fats because they do not play a healthy role in the body and they are associated with an increased risk of heart disease, whereas monounsaturated fats and the omega-3 and omega-6 sources of polyunsaturated fats are essential fats because they have a positive health role to play in the body. Regardless of whether they are essential or non-essential fats they all provide a rich source of energy. See Step Three for more details about dietary fats.

WATER

Water is the most overlooked nutrient in our diet – it forms about 60% of our total weight and is involved in every single chemical reaction in the body. If we don't get enough water we are not providing the right environment for our bodies to perform effectively. It is very important to drink at least eight glasses of water a day – it really does impact how you feel and how your body works. See Step Two for more details.

...AND ALCOHOL

While alcohol is not strictly a food group in its own right it does deserve a special mention as it is such a pleasurable part of our daily lives. It is vital however that we understand the role it plays in the body and how it constrains long-term fat loss and weight management. Alcohol does supply us with a source of energy but it is not a nutrient as it is not necessary for life and it is harmful to health when consumed in excess. See Step Two for more about this.

GETTING THE BALANCE RIGHT

For your diet to be balanced you need to eat a variety of foods from each food group – the various Body Blitz steps will go into this in more detail. Carbohydrates should form the backbone of your diet, specifically fruit and vegetables and starchy whole-grains. However, don't fall into the trap of eating too many whole-grain starches in the belief that because they are low in fat you can eat more – they may be low in fat but they still contain calories! Proteins should be consumed in a smaller volume and fats should make up the smallest part of your diet.

Most foods contain a variety of protein, fat and carbohydrate, although the combination can vary greatly from one food to another. Hence we tend to define a food by its main food group. If you consume excess calories from *any* of these food groups – not just fat – you will gain weight and body fat. Whilst some of the nutrients have specific jobs to do, once these jobs have been done any excess calories will simply be stored as fat within our fat cells.

Each of these food groups will provide an energy or calorie value to the body. Carbohydrate and protein provide 4 calories per gram, fat provides 9 calories per gram and alcohol provides 7 calories per gram. So we don't have to be an Einstein to realize that we need to look at the composition of the foods we eat as well as the total number of calories we are consuming if we want to control weight and body fat levels.

Unfortunately, there are no miracle foods to ensure weight loss. It is the whole picture of what we eat that is important for our health, weight and body fat. The Body Blitz Plan will show you that with a little knowledge you can eat whatever you want and still realize your weight and body fat goals.

THE BASIC NUTRIENTS

NUTRIENT	WHAT IS IT?	TYPICAL EXAMPLES	CALORIES PER GRAM
Carbohydrates	fruit	apples, oranges, pears	4 N.B. fruit and vegetables have a high water content so the calories per weight is kept low
	vegetables	tomatoes, carrots, kale	4
	starches	bread, pasta, rice, potatoes	4
	processed sugars	honey, syrup, jams	4

FUNCTION IN BODY	WHEN/HOW MUCH DO WE NEED?	BODY BLITZ COMMENTS
provides essential minerals and vitamins	Minimum 5 portions fruit and vegetables a day *(see Step 1 for more about this)*. Spread out fruit and vegetable intake throughout day to avoid gastro discomfort.	Most people fall short of quota.
provides essential minerals and vitamins	Minimum 5 portions fruit and vegetables a day *(see Step 1)*.	Most people fall short of quota.
good source of fuel for the body to use during the day	3–4 servings a day. Keep to breakfast and lunch to match energy demands and energy delivery. Avoid in evening meal.	Most people mistakenly eat too much when trying to lose weight. Comfort eating of these starchy carbohydrates increases overall calorie intake leading to weight and body fat gain.
provides instant energy into the bloodstream causing the blood sugars to rise and then sharply fall	Keep to absolute minimum. Obtain sugars from natural fruit sources.	The 4–6 p.m. time zone – the quick sugar fix craving increases intake of these simple sugars. Avoid the Vitamin J(unk) diet.

THE BASIC NUTRIENTS

NUTRIENT	WHAT IS IT?	TYPICAL EXAMPLES	CALORIES PER GRAM
Protein	dairy products	milk, cheese, eggs, yoghurt	4
	meat, fish, pulses	salmon, cod, chicken, beans, nuts	4
Fats	essential	polyunsaturated fats found in vegetable oils and fish oils (in cold water oily fish); monounsaturated fats found in olive oil, rapeseed oil etc.	9
	non-essential	saturated fats such as cheese, cream; lard; trans fats found in margarine, processed foods etc.	9
Water		tap, mineral water (either still or sparkling)	0
Alcohol Note: although alcohol provides us with energy it is not a nutrient as it is not necessary for life		all wine, liquor, beer	7

FUNCTION IN BODY	WHEN/HOW MUCH DO WE NEED?	BODY BLITZ COMMENTS
repairs vital cells in the body, source of calcium	Try to have a serving of protein at each meal.	Don't eat too much. Be wary of high fat content.
repairs vital cells in the body	Try to have a serving of protein at each meal.	Eating protein at lunchtime with an equal amount of starch will boost afternoon concentration powers.
helps decrease blood cholesterol levels and prevent heart disease	This should form the majority of your fat sources.	Keep visible fats to a minimum and eat 3 servings of oily fish a week.
potentially increases furring of blood vessels	Keep to a minimum.	Found in a lot of processed foods, especially snacks.
vital for all metabolic responses in the body	Minimum of 2 litres a day.	Organize yourself to drink throughout the day.
1–2 units of alcohol per day is thought to have protective effect on heart	Spread consumption of 10 units throughout week.	Avoid overindulging in social situations.

THE LOW-DOWN ON BODY FAT

So why do we have body fat and how can Body Blitz help us get rid of it? Whether we like it or not we all have fat in our bodies. Each one of us is born with 23 billion fat cells and each of these fat cells has the ability to get bigger and bigger, as well as smaller and smaller. A certain amount of fat is important for our bodies as it gives us shape, warmth and insulation – the problem comes when we start to store too much fat in the body from overeating and under activity.

It is inevitable as we get older we are going to lay down more body fat as our body's metabolism changes. To combat this we need to establish nutritional and exercise strategies to minimize body fat gain and improve our overall health. Fat cells do not disappear but the actual amount of fat in the cells can decrease and increase dependent upon how well we eat and how much exercise we take. The Body Blitz Plan provides you with all the strategies you need to lose body fat and weight – and keep it off for good!

HOW CAN WE DECREASE THE SIZE OF OUR FAT CELLS?

Unfortunately, if we are consuming more calories than we are expending our fat cells will get bigger and bigger. Although fat cells do not generally divide and increase in numbers, if we eat excessively and gain a significant amount of weight (40–50 pounds) then our fat cells will get bigger and divide and it is likely that the body fat gained at this time will pose more of a problem to shift. While this may seem depressing it helps explain why sometimes we look at friends and they appear to have dropped the weight effortlessly, while our own efforts seem to require a lot more persistence. Appreciating this will allow you to approach your Body Blitz Plan with a realistic picture of what you can achieve long-term.

The most effective way to decrease the size of your fat cells is to reduce your weekly intake of calories. This can be achieved through a combination of sensible nutrition and physical activity (see Steps One to Five for specific strategies). For fat cells to get smaller we need to create a calorie deficit of 3,500 calories per week. At first sight this figure can appear alarming, however the trick to effective body fat loss is to ensure that the calorie deficit is achieved slowly and consistently. Spreading the 3,500 over seven days means you are aiming for a decrease of 500 calories each day from your normal daily calorie range. If you split these 500 calories between **accumulated physical activities, structured exercise** and the nutritional strategies in the Body Blitz Plan, the figure becomes a lot more manageable. As we go through the book you will see how you can achieve this calorie deficit effectively, while continuing to live your life to the full. Different lifestyle constraints will mean that more emphasis will be placed on the different strategies at different times.

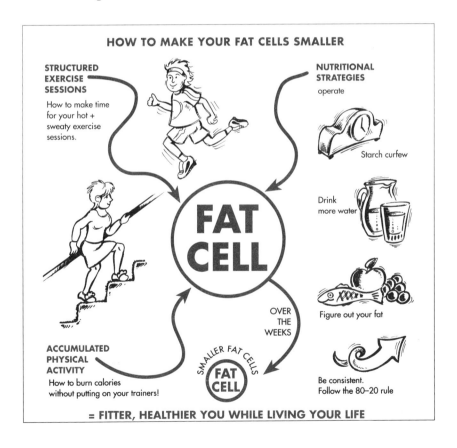

HOW TO MAKE YOUR FAT CELLS SMALLER

STRUCTURED EXERCISE SESSIONS
How to make time for your hot + sweaty exercise sessions.

NUTRITIONAL STRATEGIES
operate

Starch curfew

Drink more water

Figure out your fat

ACCUMULATED PHYSICAL ACTIVITY
How to burn calories without putting on your trainers!

FAT CELL

OVER THE WEEKS

SMALLER FAT CELLS
FAT CELL

Be consistent. Follow the 80–20 rule

= FITTER, HEALTHIER YOU WHILE LIVING YOUR LIFE

WAYS TO SAVE 500 CALORIES A DAY

Accumulated physical activity: Walk to post office rather than drive, take the stairs at work, walk up the escalators. Saves you: 100 calories

Structured exercise: Power walk for one mile. Saves you: 100 calories

Nutrition: Operate starch curfew in evening meal. Replace a portion of pasta with two portions of extra vegetables. Saves you: 200 calories

Replace mid-afternoon snack of 2 slices of bread and jam with an apple. Saves you: 100 calories.

WHY DO WE GAIN WEIGHT FASTER AS WE GET OLDER?

As we get older we actually start to lay down more body fat. This is due to several factors:

1. METABOLIC RATE

After the age of 30 if we are inactive we actually start to lose muscle mass at a rate of ⅓–½ pound every two years. So if you weighed 10 stone at the age of 20 and you still weigh 10 stone at the age of 50, yet you have gone up two clothes sizes and you do not exercise – quite simply, you have lost muscle mass and gained body fat. As the body fat takes up more space, your clothes become tighter and your clothes size goes up. Muscle is metabolically active which means that it burns calories. So if we start to lose muscle mass we actually require less calories to do our everyday tasks. Long-term this means we can potentially be consuming the same number of calories at the age of 20 as at the age of 50 but when we are 50 these calories are not burnt off and we are more prone to laying down body fat. This puts our health at risk and we become frustrated with our shape and fitness.

2. HORMONES

As women start to approach the menopause we enter a stage known as peri menopause – at this time there is a change in our hormones, which may actually encourage our bodies to lay down more body fat.

3. STRESS

Yes, stress does make us fat! When we are experiencing long periods of chronic stress such as overwork, or emotional stresses such as a loss of a partner or moving home, there is a change in our metabolism that encourages increased secretion of the hormone cortisol. If this is left unchecked for long periods of time it encourages body fat to be laid down around our midriffs. Research has shown that storing body fat here actually puts us at a greater risk of heart disease.

Whilst this all may seem a little depressing, the best possible course of action you can take is also the most accessible and cheapest – get active! Taking **structured exercise** sessions and **accumulating physical activity** during the day has both a positive and immediate impact on your health and ability to control your weight. See Step Four for more about this.

WHY DO SOME PEOPLE LOSE BODY FAT FASTER THAN OTHERS?

Not everyone will lose weight and body fat at the same rate. We are all different, and there are several factors that can affect our rate of weight and body fat loss.

These include:

1. Your existing metabolic rate
2. Your dieting history
3. Your exercise history
4. Your existing eating patterns
5. Your existing activity patterns

1. YOUR EXISTING METABOLIC RATE

As we have just discussed, our muscle mass starts to decrease as we get older and our metabolic rate tends to slow down, which means we burn fewer calories. Imagine you are 20 years old and you are sitting in a chair, and now imagine you are 50 years old sitting in a chair. Even though you are doing exactly the same everyday activity, if you have not kept up your muscle mass between the ages of 20 and 50 you will be burning less calories sitting still at the age of 50 than sitting still at the age of 20!

Action: Invest in physical activity now! Step Four of the Body Blitz Plan will help you boost your metabolic rate through **structured exercise** sessions.

2. YOUR DIETING HISTORY

If you are a seasoned dieter and you religiously try every diet on the market and have experienced weight gain/weight loss again and again – long-term it will be harder to lose weight effectively. You may already have experienced this. For example, every January you may have a favourite diet that gives you great results – well, it did the first couple of times you did it and now you are experiencing frustration as the scales are not giving you the results you want. This is because as the body is continually put through phases of excess and deficit there comes a time when our metabolism may stop working effectively and instead of losing weight we can actually increase the amount of body fat we have.

Action: Stabilize your calorie and fat intake now. Step Five of the Body Blitz Plan will show you how to **be consistent** with your nutrient intake whilst still continuing to live life to the full.

3. YOUR EXERCISE HISTORY

To lose weight and body fat you need to exercise regularly. If you were active when you were younger you will be at an advantage as muscles have a memory – this means that even if you are not exercising now the muscles will be able to respond more effectively and quickly to exercise once you do start. But even if you were not active when you were younger, it is never too late to start. Becoming active now and staying active will help you realize your fat loss goals as well as have an immediate protective effect on your health.

Action: Start being active today. Step Four of the Body Blitz Plan will show you how to increase your **accumulated physical activity** levels.

4. YOUR EXISTING EATING PATTERNS

Quite simply, the more erratic our eating patterns the harder it is to lose weight, and the longer you have had erratic eating patterns the more frustration you are likely to experience trying to lose weight. The body actually balances itself out over seven to eight days; however, in those seven to eight days if you have overeaten one day and then starved yourself the next in an attempt to make up for the excesses, the body will rebel and you will not lose weight and body fat.

To lose body fat, and for us to actually see a difference in the shape of our bodies, we need to eat a healthy and balanced diet and be consistent about it.

Action: Apply the **starch curfew** and cut your intake of fat – and **be consistent**! Steps One, Three and Five will put you in control of your diet no matter what the situation.

5. YOUR EXISTING ACTIVITY PATTERNS

If you are reading this and thinking, but I already exercise and go to the gym and I am active during my day but still I'm not losing weight, you may be experiencing frustration because:

- You do not have enough variety in your exercise programme and your body has become complacent at always doing the same thing.
- You are not working hard enough at your daily activity so you are not putting your body under enough physiological strain to increase your fitness.

Action: Complete the **activity audit** in Step Four and work out your exertion rates. This will give you a better picture of how you can expend your energy effectively.

WHERE DO WE STORE OUR BODY FAT?

Have you ever wondered why some of us seem to store all our body fat on our hips and thighs and some of us tend to have long lean arms and legs but store more of our body fat around our midriffs? This distribution of fat is associated directly to two main hormones in the body. These hormones, lipoprotein lipase LPL and hormone sensitive lipase HSL, directly affect whether we store fat or encourage it to be distributed in the blood and then burnt off. LPL tends to encourage fat storage and HSL tends to encourage fat to be burnt off. The amount of LPL and HSL we have tends to vary between men and women, individuals and areas of the body.

Men tend to have more LPL in the belly and less HSL in the lower hip area. This creates the more pronounced apple shape we see in overweight men, with more body fat distributed around the belly. Women tend to have more LPL in the hips and back of the arms and less HSL in the upper body. This classically creates more of our traditional pear shape. When women lose weight we generally still have more LPL in the hips so still have a pear shape.

So the challenge for us is to try and create more HSL and one of the best ways to do this is with EXERCISE. Weight-bearing aerobic exercise such as brisk walking, jogging and aerobics is the best form of exercise to choose. Swimming, even though it is an aerobic activity, has shown to be less effective for weight loss as it is non-weight bearing so it is not so effective in burning off calories. In addition, swimming increases LPL, which has the effect of decreasing our core temperature, which in turn can stimulate us to eat more.

The Body Blitz Plan will help you reduce your weight and body fat and boost your confidence to put you in control long-term. It is important to understand however that due to your own individual makeup your body will have an optimum shape it naturally wants to be. The Body Blitz Plan does not promise you false results but it will help you shape, tone and improve the overall appearance of your body – and it will help you lose weight and body fat and keep it off for good!

WHY IS MEASURING BODY FAT IMPORTANT?

When we stand on weighing scales we are actually measuring our total body weight which is made up of muscle tissue (also known as muscle mass or fat-free mass) and fat tissue (also known as fat mass). Muscle is denser than body fat, so if you took a pound of muscle and you took a pound of fat, the pound of fat would take up a lot more space. It is the amount of fat that we have in our bodies that actually affects our body shape and health. The reading we receive from traditional bathroom scales tells us what the total amount of our body weight is – body fat *and* muscle (and other tissue such as bone) – but it does not tell us how much fat we actually have. It is this excess body fat that is associated with heart disease, high blood pressure, diabetes and certain types of cancer. By measuring our body fat not only are we monitoring how much of our weight is actually fat but it also gives us an indicator of our health status. Monitoring our percentage body fat actually allows us to impact our health by ensuring we lose body fat as opposed to muscle mass.

Studies have shown that with very low calorie diets, the body will actually lose muscle mass and keep hold of body fat. This means that with some 'diets' you may actually increase the amount of body fat you have!

HOW CAN I MEASURE HOW MUCH BODY FAT I HAVE?

Body fat can be measured in a number of ways. One method is with **skin fold calipers**. The skin folds are generally taken at four sites around the body.

Possibly the most convenient and accurate method however is with body fat monitors. Constructed as a set of bathroom weighing scales, by entering your height and sex and standing on the scales, a safe technique known as bioelectrical impedance analysis will determine your percentage body fat. Replacing bathroom scales with body fat monitors will give a true idea of what is happening inside you – this way you get to see a complete picture of your total body weight, muscle mass and fat mass. Body fat monitors are now available from a wide range of outlets.

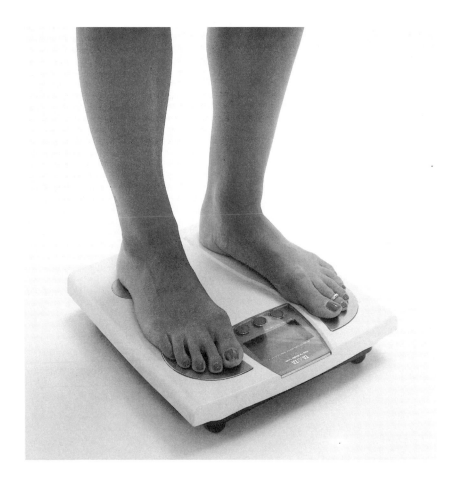

HOW MUCH BODY FAT SHOULD WE HAVE?

We all need to have body fat. Too little and we run the risk of decreased fertility
and the onset of amenorrhea, a condition where the female periods stop. Too
much body fat is associated with an increased risk of heart disease, hypertension,
diabetes and some cancers. So what exactly are the healthy ranges? The figures
shown opposite are broadly accepted as the ideal percentages for body fat.

Sex	Age 18–39 years	Age 40–59 years	Age 60+ years
Males	8%–20%	11%–22%	13%–25%
Females	21%–33%	23%–34%	24%–36%

Source: European Congress of Obesity, 1999

WHAT FAT-LOSS TARGET SHOULD WE AIM FOR?

Changing body fat does take time but the benefits you see will be long-term. A two-to-four percent decrease in body fat over a ten-week period is a sensible and realistic target. Although this may not sound a lot, in real terms this will represent a two-to-four percent decrease in the amount of fat your body is actually carrying with you day in and day out.

RECORDING YOUR PROGRESS

It is good to keep a record of how much body fat you are losing each week so you can see how much progress you are making. Here is what you do:

- Weigh yourself and establish your percentage body fat (either with a body fat monitor or with skin fold calipers), or if this is not possible then record your weight and tape measurements only.
- Using a tape measure, establish your waist measurement (measure around narrowest part of midriff), your belly button measurement (measure around midriff over belly button) and hip measurement.
- Record these measurements at the same time each week.

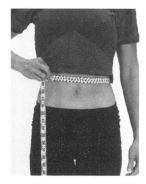 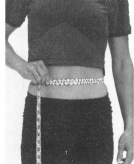 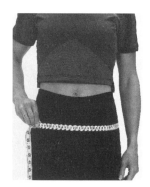

MEASURING YOURSELF

Body Blitz Progress Chart

DATE	WEIGHT	BODY FAT PERCENTAGE	WAIST MEASUREMENT	BELLY BUTTON MEASUREMENT	HIP MEASUREMENT
Week One					
Week Two					
Week Three					
Week Four					
Week Five					
Week Six					

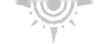

FACTORS DETERMINING YOUR SUCCESS

YOUR WILLPOWER

The strength of your willpower is an important factor in how successful you will be at realizing your weight and body fat goals. Generally an individual's willpower is at its weakest towards the end of the day – perhaps we feel tired or our blood sugars are low. This means that we tend to have less control of our actions at this time and are more likely to overeat or eat all the inappropriate foods. If you are constantly tired and struggling with your weight, you may well be building up extra calories at the end of the day that do not get burnt off. Here are a few questions for you to think about:

1. When am I most physically active?
   - between seven a.m. to six p.m.
   - after six p.m. to bedtime

2. When do I consume the majority of my food?
   - between seven a.m. to six p.m.
   - after six p.m. to bedtime

3. When is my willpower at its strongest?
   - first thing in the morning
   - midday
   - mid-afternoon
   - evening

Invariably what happens is there is a mismatch between when we need to receive energy from our food and when we are expending energy through our everyday activities. The chart below shows that generally we expend most energy between seven a.m. in the morning and six p.m. in the evening. However, we actually receive the vast majority of our energy from food after six p.m. when we are less active. While some studies suggest that it makes no difference whether your calories from food are consumed during the day or all at night, what these studies fail to take into account is our own personal willpower. At the end of the day when we are tired, especially when we have not eaten much during the day, willpower will be low and we will be much more likely to overeat. This means long-term there is a situation where at the end of each day there is actually a build of excess calories which we are not burning off prior to going to bed – and these calories are being laid down in the fat cells as additional body fat. The Body Blitz Plan will show you how to make the right food choices at the right time of the day, so you receive energy when you need it and you don't end up with a build up of excess calories before you go to bed.

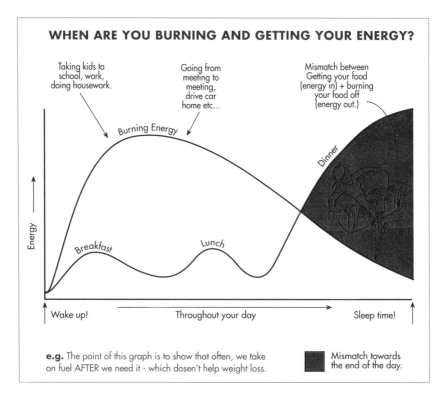

WHEN ARE YOU BURNING AND GETTING YOUR ENERGY?

Taking kids to school, work, doing housework.

Going from meeting to meeting, drive car home etc...

Mismatch between Getting your food (energy in) + burning your food off (energy out.)

Burning Energy

Dinner

Breakfast

Lunch

Energy

Wake up!   Throughout your day   Sleep time!

e.g. The point of this graph is to show that often, we take on fuel AFTER we need it - which dosen't help weight loss.

Mismatch towards the end of the day.

YOUR ATTITUDE TO FOOD

What we were introduced to as a child defines our relationship with food in later life. If you ate a lot of sugar and sweet things as you were growing up and your diet did not include a variety of tastes, it is likely you now crave calorie-dense sweet foods rather than savoury foods. Maybe your mother used to say to you, 'You must finish everything on your plate?', and now you *always* finish everything on your plate thinking it is rude to leave even a morsel. Or alternatively you had a mother who actively encouraged you not to eat certain foods or not to overeat as it would only make you fat. Or maybe you had a mother who was always on a diet and never ate the same food as the rest of the family. Our mums are great but we need to be aware of how their attitude to food impacts our attitude to food in later life. These attitudes have had a long time to be grooved and they will take a long time to diminish. The Body Blitz Plan will help you reevaluate your relationship with food, showing you how to draw up a sensible eating plan that will help you realize your weight and body fat goals as well as providing a positive health message for your children.

YOUR MOTIVATION

What is your motivation to lose weight? Is it to squeeze into that little black dress for a certain event or is it about looking better for a significant A.N. Other. Whatever your motivation you need to identify it and shift it from an external motivation such as an important event to an internal one such as wanting to feel more in control of your eating habits, have more energy and feel better about yourself. All of which translates into a strategy that you can incorporate and build on to achieve your long-term weight and body fat goals. Think about this: what we weigh in seven years will not be determined by what we do for the next seven hours or the next seven days but by how well we eat and how physically active we are over the next seven years. Establishing a strategy and following an action plan that you can keep to will be crucial – the Body Blitz Plan will show you how to do this. Seeing results is a huge motivation and with a little effort that motivation can be your driving force.

YOUR FRIENDS

Early on in your Body Blitz Plan you need to establish who are going to be saboteurs and supporters of your efforts. Within your circle of friends and family there will be individuals who will encourage you and help you with your efforts. It is also likely there will be individuals who either intentionally or unintentionally try to hinder your efforts – this may be because your efforts and seeing you look and feel better makes them feel less comfortable or they are just genuinely unaware of their intentions. Identifying who are your diet friends or foes will help you to apply the Body Blitz strategies more effectively and successfully.

YOUR PERSONALIZED BODY BLITZ PLAN

As you work through the book you will be able to build up your own personal Body Blitz Plan, using the nutritional and exercise strategies to help you realize your goals. It is important to understand that there is no one diet that works for everyone; instead Body Blitz contains strategies that accommodate a series of scenarios for a number of different types of people with different lifestyle constraints (as detailed below). Have a read through and see which one relates most closely to you. The Body Blitz Plan will also allow you to accommodate these different roles as your life changes.

- **BUSY MUM:** frantic kids, juggling school runs, part-time job and running a home, high domestic stress levels, children's meal times, lack of sleep with baby leads to reduced energy levels, no time for herself, food grabbed on the run.

- **BUSINESS WOMAN:** entertains with work, lunches and dines out frequently, high commercial stress levels, eats snacks for quick energy fixes, no time to think about sensible eating and exercise.

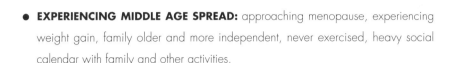

● **EXPERIENCING MIDDLE AGE SPREAD:** approaching menopause, experiencing weight gain, family older and more independent, never exercised, heavy social calendar with family and other activities.

● **GIRL ABOUT TOWN:** socializes a lot, breakfast and lunch often grabbed on the run, sees friends and eats out several times a week, alcohol can feature prominently in the social calendar.

● **SEASONED DIETER:** tried every diet around, routinely loses weight and then gains it back, more recently finding it harder to shift the weight and body fat.

Throughout the book you will find nutritional and exercise strategies for each individual – once you have identified which type relates most closely to you, you will be able to use the guidelines offered to design your own personal exercise and fitness plan that fits in with your life, just the way it is.

A FINAL WORD

So remember, the Body Blitz Plan is about being the best you can be whilst still living the life you wish to live. Yes, it does require a little bit of effort but you don't have to make any big sacrifices or radical changes to your lifestyle to get the results you want – all you need to do is apply the five steps in the Body Blitz Plan (see Part II) and you will achieve your weight and fat loss goals not just for now, but for the future too.

Body Blitz Active Action Points:

- Write a list of the main obstacles to you achieving your fat loss goals – try to be as specific as possible, for example, mid-morning coffee break with work colleagues or tea time with the kids when you are starving yourself.

- Make a commitment today to make one small change in your daily activities that you will keep up for the next six weeks. For example, say no to coffee in your mid-morning coffee break and have a cup of herbal tea instead. Remember, every small change you make will take you one step further towards achieving your fat loss goals.

PART II: 5-STEP BODY BLITZ PLAN TO PERMANENT FAT LOSS!

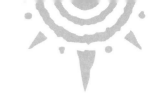

CHAPTER THREE

Step 1: The Starch Curfew – Cut your carbs after 5 p.m.

We all know we have to steer clear of a diet that contains too much fat and we feel proud of ourselves if we have said no to chocolate or ice-cream. So why are we still struggling with our weight and body fat? These days one of the most common reasons for our weight loss frustrations is that we have come to rely on low-fat starches and we are lulled into a false sense of low-fat security thinking we can eat more of these foods. A high consumption of starch however can provide more calories than we need. If we are unable to burn off these calories so they become stored as fat, all of which leads to the scales and belt notches not moving in the direction we want.

So the first step of the Body Blitz Plan is to operate the **starch curfew**. In this chapter you'll learn all about the role of starch and its impact on the body and how to:

- Use the **starch curfew** – no starches after 5 p.m.
- Adapt your meals to make sure you get the right range of nutrients and don't eat too much starch.
- Make good food choices when you are faced with a situation where there is starch on the menu and you are not allowed to eat it.

Body Blitz Must Dos

The two keys to making carbohydrates work for you are:

1. Operate the **starch curfew** to decrease total calorie intake.
2. Consume five portions of fruit and vegetables a day.

WHAT IS THE STARCH CURFEW?

As we discussed in *The Body Blitz Lifestyle* chapter starch, processed sugars and fruit and vegetables are all carbohydrates. The starch foods are potatoes, bread, rice, pasta and cereals, all of which provide a good source of fuel for the body to use during the day.

The **starch curfew** means you can eat starch at breakfast, lunch and in your mid-afternoon snack but you are not allowed to eat it after five p.m. The evening meal now comprises of protein, fruit and vegetables, low-fat dairy products and essential fats. It is a strategy that allows you to get the right balance of calories and nutrients at the right time in the day. At first this may seem a little difficult to apply but you will soon feel the huge benefits in your energy levels and you'll certainly appreciate the change in your body shape as you become less bloated.

The **starch curfew** however is not just about saying no to starches after five p.m. – it is about getting the right balance of your overall intake of starches and nutrients throughout the day. For example you may be consuming too many calories from starch foods which are contributing to your body fat, so once you reduce the amount of starch you eat you will you lose weight and body fat. Also, you will be more in control of your energy levels as you will be eating the right amount of starch at the right time for optimum energy. We will talk more about this later in the chapter.

ARE YOU A CARBO COMFORT-EATER?

Answer the questions in the following quiz to find out if you are prone to overeating on comfort starches such as bread, pasta, rice and potatoes.

1. Do you tend to snack on?

    a. bread and comfort carbohydrates such as cakes and chocolate
    b. fruit and vegetables

2. Do you munch bread with each meal?

    a. yes
    b. no

3. Do you feel lethargic in the afternoons?

    a. yes
    b. no

4. Do you eat most of your calories at the end of your day?

    a. yes
    b. no

5. Do you crave carbohydrates?

    a. yes
    b. no

6. Do you experience swings in your energy and mood?

    a. yes
    b. no

7. Do you find it difficult to stop eating comfort starches like biscuits, bread and pasta?

a. yes

b. no

If you answered:

MAINLY A'S:

You are sensitive to comfort carbohydrates, specifically the comfort foods that are starch-based. You probably have a tendency to eat more of these foods than is appropriate and this causes you to feel lethargic and out of control.

Action: Operate the **starch curfew** and use the **starch-free zone** when faced with an excess starch situation.

MAINLY B'S:

You are less prone to overindulging on carbohydrates. If you experience problems with your weight it may be due to excess calories consumed through carbohydrates or an imbalance in your nutrient intake.

Action: Introduce the **starch curfew** as a tool to control calorie intake.

WATCH THOSE CALORIES!

I developed the **starch curfew** concept as a nutritional diet tool when I realized a number of my weight management clients were experiencing initial weight and body fat loss but then they were reaching a plateau with their weight loss and their efforts seemed to go no further. This seemed to be a recurring theme not just with my clients but also with other people's initial weight loss success stories.

My clients were all very efficient at decreasing the overall fat in their diets, but because their focus was on fat their attention slipped from their carbohydrate intake – specifically bread, pasta, rice, potatoes and cereal were all being over-consumed and often in the evening as opposed to during the day when our body may burn these nutrients more effectively. A typical daily food intake looked something like this:

Breakfast:	cereal with skimmed milk and banana
Lunch:	large jacket potato with sweet corn, one banana
Snack:	chunk of bread with fruit jam
Dinner:	pasta with homemade tomato sauce, brown bread roll

Now at first glance this seems to be a pretty healthy diet and to a certain extent it is, however what it lacks is essential fats, a minimum of five portions of fruit and vegetables, protein and suitable portion sizes. The classic mistake is that too many calories were being consumed. So while fat intake was decreased and in fact very low, the consumption of calories through starches was increasing.

Total calorie intake does count. So while we may be very good at reducing the amount of fat in our diet, if the total number of calories consumed is higher than the amount of calories being burnt off through exercise and activity, then weight gain can actually occur regardless that the source of calories were 'fat-free'.

Have a look at the table below to see the calorie content of some typical starch foods – this will help you to see how excess calories from starch might be contributing to your body fat.

Calorie Content of Starch Foods

Food	Calorie Value
1 large slice wholemeal bread	100
pasta (100g dry weight)	405
rice (100g dry weight)	400
1 jacket potato (200g raw weight)	160
1 bagel	225
1 croissant	295
1 large pitta	180
1 hot cross bun	190
bowl of bran flakes (40g)	147
1 naan bread	450
4 roast potatoes (200g)	340
1 burger bun	140
slice of focaccia bread	160
1 crumpet	80

WHAT ARE THE BENEFITS OF USING THE STARCH CURFEW?

As I explained at the beginning of the chapter, you can eat starch in moderation at breakfast, lunch and in your mid-afternoon snack but you cannot eat it in your evening meal. By operating the **starch curfew** you will:

- Help decrease your overall calorie intake.
- Help decrease your overall starch intake. Excess starch stimulates the production of serotonin in the brain, which can make us feel more sluggish. This in turn directly stimulates us to reach for the instant high of a sugar fix such as chocolate, sugary sweet cakes, biscuits and processed snacks.

- Beat your sugar cravings. Eating the right amounts of protein and starch at lunchtime will fuel you with energy and brainpower all afternoon.

Serotonin and Dopamine

Too great a dependence on starchy carbohydrates, whilst vital for storing energy in our muscles, can make us feel lethargic due to the production of the brain neurotransmitter serotonin. This is why we often experience a slump of energy immediately after our lunch – we have consumed too many starches at lunchtime. Conversely, proteins consumed in the right amount increases the release of the hormone-like substance dopamine, which makes us feel more alert, increases our ability to concentrate and helps to regulate our mood.

WHY DOES THE STARCH CURFEW WORK?

The **starch curfew** works because:

1. By eating your starch at breakfast and lunch, it means you consume more energy-providing nutrients during the day. This will give you more physical and mental energy to meet the daily demands and pleasures of life.
2. It allows you to have a lighter meal in the evening based on protein and fruit and vegetables. This helps you achieve a healthier balance of nutrients, as without the presence of bread, pasta, rice, grains and potatoes you will really need to fill up on fruit and vegetables.
3. Eating less in the evening will make you hungry for a lovely healthy breakfast – this will fuel you with energy right through the day.

THE LOW-DOWN ON CARBOHYDRATES

SHOULD WE EAT CARBOHYDRATES?

Yes, carbohydrates form the backbone of our diet. Fruit and vegetables should be eaten at each meal; starches can be eaten at breakfast and lunch but not in your evening meal, and processed sugars should be kept to an absolute minimum. It is important to remember that the different types of carbohydrates are treated by the body in different ways. The trick to successful weight and body fat loss is to make sure you are eating the right carbohydrates at the right time of the day, so your body receives the right type of carbohydrate when it needs it. This will help you achieve and maintain your weight and body fat goals, you will have more energy during the day, and most importantly, you will minimize your hunger pangs.

To help you understand how the **starch curfew** works, the table below shows you when to eat *what* carbohydrate foods for optimum energy and weight loss.

Carbohydrates	Food Examples	When to Eat
starches	all breads, pasta, rice, potatoes, sweet potatoes, cereal, oats, bulgur wheat, millet	breakfast, lunch and mid-afternoon snack – you are not allowed to consume in mid-morning snack or after 5 p.m.
fruit	apples, nectarines, melons, grapes	all meals and snacks, especially in evening meal
vegetables	peppers, kale, carrots, broccoli	all meals and snacks, especially in evening meal
processed sugars	sweets, chocolates, cakes, biscuits	minimal consumption

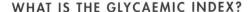

WHAT IS THE GLYCAEMIC INDEX?

Traditionally carbohydrate foods, which provide the main fuel base for our bodies, are classified as simple or complex carbohydrates. Simple carbohydrates such as sugars, some fruits, cakes and biscuits provide a quick increase in blood glucose levels whilst complex carbohydrates such as brown rice, porridge oats and wholegrains raise blood glucose at a slower rate and keep blood glucose levels more stable for longer. The rate at which our blood sugars change with eating different types of carbohydrates is called the glycaemic index (GI). The concept of GI carbohydrates is fairly new and is particularly recommended for individuals who may be sensitive to swings in energy. Here is a table to help you assess the GI of the carbohydrate foods you eat. Pure sugar receives a value of 100, and other sugary foods and starches are compared to that. Later in the chapter, to help you optimise your energy levels, we'll look at when it is best to eat which GI carbohydrates.

Glycaemic Index Carbohydrates

Glycaemic Index Rating	Food
100	sugar
80 – 90	carrots, cornflakes, honey, parsnips, potatoes
70 – 79	wholewheat bread, white rice
60 – 69	bananas, white bread, raisins, brown rice
50 – 59	porridge oats, frozen peas, pasta, sweet potatoes
below 50	oranges, orange juice, dried peas, apples, fructose

IS IT OKAY TO GRAB A QUICK SUGAR FIX?

Sugar gives us an instant release of energy, which is then followed by an energy low. When we consume a large concentrated form of sugar, such as a slice of chocolate cake or a commercially-made muffin, the hormone insulin reacts to the elevated blood glucose levels and transfers the sugar from the blood into the cells. This response is so effective that the body can decrease the blood sugar levels very effectively. This in turn creates a feeling of further tiredness, lack of energy and increased appetite about 90 minutes after you had your first chocolate fix. So while sugar has a role to play in the diet, its ability to provide a quick instant energy boost is short-lived and can create a roller-coaster of high and low blood sugar levels, which sends us craving more sugar as well as for some of us causing depression and continued fatigue. So instead of relying on sugar from sweets we need to rely more on the natural sources of sugars from fruit and vegetables to stabilise our blood sugar levels.

HOW MUCH FRUIT AND VEGETABLES SHOULD WE EAT?

The World Health Organization recommends we eat at least five portions of fruit and vegetables a day. But what exactly is one portion? Unfortunately the slice of tomato in our sandwich does not equal a portion! And sorry potatoes do not count, as they are a starch.

Here are some examples of the amount of fruit and vegetables in one portion:

• apple, orange or banana	1 fruit
• very large fruit e.g. melon, pineapple	1 large slice
• small fruits e.g. plums, kiwi, satsuma	2 fruit
• raspberries, strawberries, grapes	1 cup
• fresh fruit salad, stewed or canned	1–1 1/2 cups
• dried fruit	1 cup
• fruit juice	1 glass (150ml)
• vegetables, raw, cooked, frozen or canned	1 cup
• salad	1 dessert bowl

Count up what you are eating now – if it is less than five portions a day, add in one more and gradually build up to five.

WHAT ABOUT FIBRE?

Fibre is the indigestible portion of carbohydrate. There are two types of fibre: soluble fibre found mainly in fruits, vegetables and in some grains, particularly oats, and insoluble fibre found mainly in the bran portion of cereal grains. Research has shown that a diet rich in soluble fibre is associated with a reduced risk of developing heart disease and diabetes, while a diet rich in insoluble fibre will help reduce cholesterol levels and is beneficial for bowel movement. No single food supplies all the soluble and insoluble fibre needed for health, so a wide variety of minimally processed, high fibre foods as included in the Body Blitz Plan are recommended. Studies linking fibre to a reduced risk of disease have investigated naturally occurring fibre-rich foods such as vegetables, fruits, beans and whole-grains. Be wary of commercialized fibre-based products such as bran muffins as these are often high in fat, sugar or salt.

EATING FOR ENERGY

The key to the **starch curfew** is to keep your energy levels up by making sure you eat the right type of carbohydrate at the right time of day. The tables below, in conjunction with the eating plans and recipes at the end of the book, will help you put the **starch curfew** into practice.

WHEN TO EAT YOUR CARBOHYDRATES

Glycaemic Index Rating	Food Examples	When to Eat	Body Blitz Comments
high GI	bread, bagel, pastry, cornflakes, potatoes, rice, parsnips, raisins, bananas, chocolate and semi-sweet biscuits	breakfast, lunch, after structured exercise session	Consuming high GI foods at breakfast can leave you feeling hungry later in the morning, so consume with some protein to offset fast release of sugars, e.g. wholemeal toast with boiled egg or have a glass of milk with your toast. Do **not** eat in your evening meal. Operate the starch curfew.
moderate GI	pasta, porridge oats, noodles, oatmeal biscuits, sweet potatoes, grapes	breakfast, lunch, after structured exercise session	If you are prone to lapses of energy mid-morning, choose a moderate GI carbohydrate for breakfast. Consume with some protein to provide slow release of energy during the day. Porridge and oatmeal are your best choices at breakfast.
low GI	most fruit and vegetables	breakfast, lunch, evening meal	Consume with protein sources for evening meal.

WHEN TO EAT YOUR STARCHES?

MEAL	CHOOSE	FOOD EXAMPLES
breakfast	a high or moderate GI source of starch with a piece of fruit	porridge made with skimmed milk, served with handful raisins and half a banana
mid-morning snack	no starch, only fruit or vegetables	a pear
lunch	a high or moderate GI source of starch with a serving of protein	open tuna salad sandwich
mid-afternoon snack	a moderate GI source of starch (though a piece of fruit or yoghurt or smoothie is a better choice as this will hydrate the body)	slice of rye bread with fruit spread
evening meal	starch curfew: **no** bread, pasta, rice, potatoes, cereal after 5 p.m. eat protein with vegetables and fruit	grilled steak with mushrooms, onions and peppers sautéed in one teaspoon of olive oil, served with large mixed green salad made with rocket, spinach, tomatoes, peppers, carrots and watercress

STARTING THE DAY RIGHT!

You can optimize your energy and put yourself in the best possible position to achieve your weight and body fat goals by starting your day with the right type of breakfast.

BREAKFAST

Starting your day with a healthy breakfast is important as it refuels your body and provides you with energy right through the day. However, you need to make sure you get the right type of breakfast to minimize hunger pangs mid-morning. Here are some examples of breakfasts which will boost your energy first thing in the morning, whilst keeping your calorie content down. A Body Blitz breakfast is a great way to start the day!

TOP 10 BREAKFASTS

The list below gives examples of breakfasts which are low in fat and nutrient-dense. They are in no particular order.

1. **PORRIDGE WITH RASPBERRIES:** 30g of porridge oats made with skimmed milk. Serve with a handful of raspberries.

2. **BOILED EGG WITH SLICE OF WHOLEMEAL TOAST:** Serve with a glass of orange juice.

3. **SUMMER FRUIT SALAD:** Large bowl of strawberries, honeydew melon and nectarines. Serve with a small handful of rolled oats and 150g pot of plain low-fat yoghurt.

4. **BRAN CEREAL WITH APRICOTS AND SULTANAS:** Mix together 30g bran cereal, 2 dried apricots and 15g sultanas and add $1/4$ pint skimmed milk. Serve with a small glass of grapefruit juice.

5. **BANANA SMOOTHIE:** 1 ripe banana (frozen), 250ml semi-skimmed milk, 1 tablespoon wheatgerm, 4 strawberries. Blend and go!

6. **RAISIN TOAST WITH SLICED PLUM:** Spread 2 slices of raisin toast with quark and top with sliced plum.

7. **SWISS MUESLI:** Soak 30g porridge oats overnight with enough water to cover. Serve with skimmed milk or low-fat live bio yoghurt and a pinch of nutmeg, sultanas and grated apple.

8. **WHOLEMEAL TOAST WITH COTTAGE CHEESE AND MARMITE:** Spread 2 slices of wholemeal toast with cottage cheese and marmite or yeast spread.

9. **POACHED EGG WITH WHOLEMEAL TOAST:** Add a dash of Worcestershire sauce for seasoning and serve with 2 slices of wholegrain toast and $1/2$ grilled tomato.

10. **CITRUS MEDLEY AND OPEN BACON SARNIE:** Segment $1/2$ orange grapefruit and $1/2$ pink grapefruit – and season with ground cinnamon. Serve with one slice of toasted soda bread with two lean grilled bacon rashers.

You will find further breakfast ideas in the *Body Blitz 14-Day Eating Plan* chapter.

GETTING IT RIGHT IN THE MIDDLE OF THE DAY!

Eating the right foods at lunchtime will fuel you with energy for the afternoon, help you avoid those mid-afternoon sugar pangs and help stabilize your calorie intake through the day. To make this work for you, you need to eat an equal amount of protein and starch in your midday meal.

WHY DO I NEED PROTEIN AT LUNCHTIME?

It is really important to eat protein at lunchtime as it increases the release of the hormone-like substance dopamine in our body. As I mentioned earlier, this is a brain transmitter which helps us to feel more alert, improves our concentration and helps regulate moods. Often we feel lethargic after lunch – this may be because we consume the wrong balance of nutrients in our midday meal. If we eat too much starch at lunchtime it increases the amount of serotonin in the brain, which may make us feel more lethargic. You need to eat protein with starch at lunchtime and preferably in the ratio of one portion of starch to one portion of protein. This means instead of having a sandwich with two pieces of bread and a ham filling (this gives a food ratio of two starch to one protein), you eat an open ham sandwich with one piece of bread (this gives a food ratio of one starch to one protein). Not only does this help to give you a better balance of nutrients, it will also save you calories.

WHAT IS A PORTION SIZE?

Have a look at the list opposite to find out how much a portion of starch and protein is. Knowing exactly how much starch and protein we are eating will help us get the food ratio right at lunchtime.

You can also visually estimate portion size for convenience. The general rule is that a portion of starch looks roughly the same size as a portion of protein. This means, for example, if you are having a jacket potato you will add a portion of cottage cheese roughly the same size as the potato. Or if you are making an open sandwich you will add a layer of protein, such as tuna or chicken, the same thickness as the slice of bread.

ONE PORTION OF STARCH EQUALS

- 1 slice regular bread
- 2 slices 'extra thin' or 'diet' bread
- $1/2$ English muffin
- $1/2$ hotdog or hamburger bun
- 1 small dinner roll
- $1/2$ cup of starchy vegetables
- $1/2$ cup of mashed potato or 1 small baked potato
- $1/2$ cup cooked cereal, pasta or rice
- 1 tortilla 6" across
- 30g cold cereal
- 4–6 crackers
- 3 cups air-popped popcorn
- 2 rice cakes or 5 mini-cakes

ONE PORTION OF PROTEIN EQUALS

Dairy
- 1 cup of skimmed milk
- $1/4$ cup semi-skimmed milk
- $3/4$ cup fruit-flavoured yoghurt
- 1 cup non-fat yoghurt
- $1/2$ cup low-fat yoghurt
- 42–56g low-fat cheese
- 30g natural cheese
- $1/2$ cup cottage cheese

Meat, Fish, Poultry and Eggs
- 84g cooked lean meat, fish or poultry
- $1/2$ cup cooked beans
- 1 medium egg

Don't Forget About the Pulses...

Pulses such as kidney, canellini and flageolot beans are an important ingredient in the Body Blitz diet. As I mentioned earlier, we define foods by their main food group – so although pulses are defined as proteins they also have a carbohydrate content. Pulses score a low GI index rating, which means that they produce a small rise in blood sugar levels, which helps us to stabilize energy levels and mood swings. Pulses are great additions to both our midday and evening meal.

TOP 10 LUNCHES

The following list shows you how to obtain the right ratio of starch and protein at lunchtime. (Note: portion size does matter!). You will find further ideas for your midday meal in the recipe section at the end of the book.

1. **OPEN SANDWICH:** 1 slice pumpernickel bread, 100g smoked salmon, 1 tablespoon low-fat yoghurt and garnish with cod roe. Serve with large spinach salad.

2. **JACKET POTATO WITH COTTAGE CHEESE:** 200g potato with 150g reduced fat cottage cheese. Serve with side salad.

3. **BROWN RICE, KIDNEY BEAN AND PEA SALAD:** 1 cup of cooked brown rice with $1/2$ cup of kidney beans and peas. Dress in balsamic vinegar dressing made with $1/2$ teaspoon olive oil.

4. **BOILED EGG:** Serve with 3 ryvitas and 2 tomatoes.

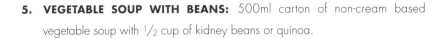

5. **VEGETABLE SOUP WITH BEANS:** 500ml carton of non-cream based vegetable soup with $^1/_2$ cup of kidney beans or quinoa.

6. **CHARGRILLED CHICKEN WRAP:** Soft flour tortilla filled with grilled, poached or roast chicken breast (no skin), sliced tomato, 2 slices of avocado, $^1/_2$ tablespoon natural yoghurt and sprinkled with fresh coriander.

7. **SUSHI:** Mixed medium sushi box (250g). Serve with a small glass of orange juice.

8. **BLT PITTA:** Wholemeal pitta bread filled with salad, 25g grilled lean back bacon (all visible fat removed), small boiled egg and a sliced tomato.

9. **SOUP WITH TOFU:** 500ml carton of commercial or home made non-cream based vegetable soup with 100g cubed tofu.

10. **PASTA SALAD:** 100g cooked pasta shapes mixed with 150g pot of low-fat cottage cheese, chopped tomato and fresh basil. Season with salt and pepper.

You will find further ideas for your midday meal in the *Eating In* and the *Body Blitz 14-Day Eating Plan* chapters in Part III.

END YOUR DAY RIGHT!

As we have already established, it is very important to eat the right foods at the end of the day. Remember, you are not allowed to eat starches after five p.m. Instead you will be eating protein, fruit and vegetables, low-fat dairy products and essential fats in your evening meal. At the end of the book there are over 20 starch-free recipes for you to choose from – they will help you to put the

starch curfew into practice and show you how easy it can be with a bit of know-how to keep your calorie intake in check.

The Body Blitz 14-day Eating Plan chapter will also give you ideas for your evening meal.

AVOIDING THE STARCHES!

What happens when the people you are with are eating starch and you can't because you are operating the starch curfew? Have a look at the table opposite to see how you can make sensible food choices when you are faced with a situation where there is starch on the menu. The starch curfew gives you the flexibility to see what other foods you can eat and enjoy aside from starch, so you can continue to enjoy *all* your social activities and you are not put in the position where everyone can see that you are on a diet.

Part III contains further advice about how to make good food choices when eating out in a variety of restaurants with cuisine from around the world. Just because you are operating the **starch curfew**, it does not mean you cannot enjoy your evening meal. In fact, you will probably be surprised at just how many delicious starch-free dishes you can choose from the menu.

THE STARCH-FREE ZONE

There will be times when the **starch curfew** is out of the question – perhaps, for example, you are going to a dinner party at a friend's house and you know it's going to be virtually impossible to go starch-free. On these occasions you can bring in the **starch-free zone**.

The **starch-free zone** means you say no to starch in your midday meal, thus freeing up your starch intake to have in your evening meal. If from time to time your lifestyle doesn't fit in with the Body Blitz Plan, don't beat yourself up about it – the Body Blitz Plan allows you to balance things out over time. We will talk more about this in Step Five and you will see how you can put the **starch-free zone** into practice in a variety of different scenarios.

Scenario	Action Points	Suggested Meal Choice
eating in a restaurant	say no to the bread basket; select a starch-free choice from the menu; request your dish to be served without the potatoes/rice etc.	Starter: smoked salmon (no bread) Main course: grilled meat or fish with salad or vegetables Dessert: try to avoid but if necessary opt for fresh fruit sorbet
eating at home by yourself or with partner	prepare evening meal with protein foods, pulses, vegetables and fruit	light chicken curry with spinach (see page 192)
eating at home with family	prepare starch-free main meal; cook starch (potatoes, rice or pasta) for rest of family	provencal-style poached chicken with vegetables (see page 193). Serve with new potatoes and bread for the family
entertaining with guests	prepare a selection of dishes that are starch-free, but serve with specialty breads, rice and pastas as an additional extra. Make the vegetables and protein the main emphasis of the dish	chicken and apricot tagine (see page 190). Serve with green salad or prawn, scallops and parma ham kebabs with parsley salad (see page 196)

BODY BLITZ SUCCESS STORIES

CAROLYN

Carolyn is a business woman who works long hours as well as leading a really hectic social life. Originally from Australia, she is determined to 'live it up' in London while she is working in England. Here is her story:

> Within eight months of arriving in London, I was experiencing substantial weight gain – this is something many foreigners suffer from having led physically active lives before arriving in the city and then sedentary lives once here. It concerned me so I attempted to lose this weight, but slowly I became extremely frustrated as I was making no progress. So I started the Body Blitz Plan and I can honestly say I felt the difference immediately. The biggest success factor for me was the starch curfew. It really helped me to stabilize my calorie intake – and at the same time it still allowed me to enjoy London and it didn't interfere with my social life.
>
> Even within four weeks I had lost eight inches off my body and I continued to lose weight. The best part is that it is not only achievable but also fun. With such positive results it gives me the encouragement to keep going. The strategies have given me a new lease of life and I feel confident that I will able to maintain it in the future.

So how did Carolyn do?

Carolyn lost fourteen pounds in body weight – this meant she had dropped two dress sizes in just nine weeks.

Carolyn's Starch Curfew Menu Makeover

Meals	Before	Now
breakfast	2 slices of toast with marmalade and butter, small glass orange juice, cup of tea	2 slices of wholemeal toast with cottage cheese and glass orange juice or Body Blitz breakfast smoothie *(see page 218)*
lunch	jacket potato with baked beans	small jacket potato with tuna and side salad
snack	a banana, thick slice of bread with fruit puree jam	an apple
dinner	pasta with tomato sauce, grated cheese and garlic bread on the side, yoghurt for dessert	150g uncooked weight of lean meat or fish, served with green salad, broccoli and carrots, yoghurt with sliced fruit for dessert

ALEXANDRA

Alexandra had fought a battle with her weight all her life – she had tried every lotion, pill and diet on the market in her endeavour to meet her weight and body fat goals. But she never seemed to achieve the results she sought in the first place and she was never able to keep the weight and body fat off. This is her story:

Thanks to the Body Blitz Plan my 'tree trunk' legs are vastly reduced for the first time in my life – and without losing weight on my face which is what has always happened in the past when I have tried to slim down. In my case, I attribute my success to eating a proper breakfast plus a sensible lunch – before Body Blitz I had three cups of coffee and nothing else till a couple of crackers with a wedge of cheese at lunchtime, so I was starving by dinnertime and would then binge on stodgy bread, potatoes and pasta. Even though I was eating my pasta with low-fat sauces, I was just eating too much of it! Now I always have porridge for breakfast (made with water and fruit), which really does release energy slowly throughout the morning and a proper lunch – either a mixed salad with some tinned salmon, pilchards or cottage cheese or an open rye bread chicken and salad sandwich.

So how did Alexandra do?

After a year of sensible eating of quite large quantities, I find I have gone down from nine stone to seven stone ten pounds without much hassle. This may sound very light but I have a very small frame and I am only five foot! Everyone says I have completely changed shape and look so well all the time (even after a night on the tiles!), so I am seriously grateful to Body Blitz and intend to keep up this lifestyle forever.

A FINAL WORD

So as we can see, the **starch curfew** is a great concept that allows you to eat the same food as your family, keep your calorie intake down, while boosting your intake of filling and healthy vegetables, pulses and fruit. You will find you have more energy throughout the day and you will wake up feeling less sluggish. So start applying the **starch curfew** now and you will soon feel the benefits whilst enjoying all your daily social activities. Don't worry if this seems a challenge at first – the recipes at the end of the book will help give you ideas and you will soon find you can adapt your meals quickly and easily, accommodating the whole family at the same time. Go on, start putting the **starch curfew** into practice today!

Body Blitz Active Action Points:

- Start operating the starch curfew – begin this week.
- Draw up menu plans either from the suggested eating plans or the recipes at the end of the book.
- Plan ahead to see when you might need to implement a starch-free zone at lunchtime.

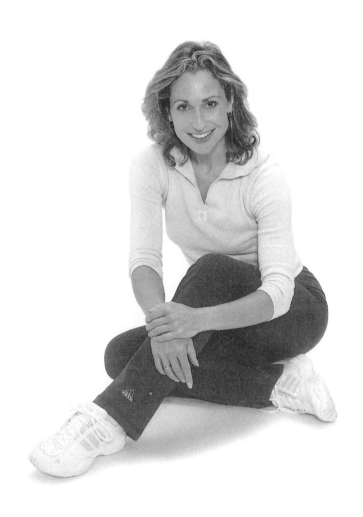

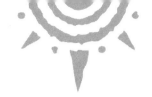

CHAPTER FOUR

Step 2: H₂O – Why more water means less fat

No natural resource is undervalued as much as water. These days most people do not drink nearly enough water. In fact, very many people never drink any at all and imagine that tea, coffee and fizzy drinks do much the same job, which they do not. It is very important to drink water to hydrate our bodies and flush out toxins and accumulated wastes from the system. If you drink less than eight glasses of water a day your body may be chronically dehydrated, you will lack energy and your brain can misinterpret this tiredness as a need to eat more food.

Feeling devoid of energy is one of the biggest challenges we face, especially when we are on a diet. So often we put a lack of energy down to not having eaten enough or slept enough, so we reach for a sugar fix for that instant energy boost. In fact, water has a greater impact on our energy levels than any other nutrient. So when we are tired we need to address how well-hydrated our body is first to ensure we are giving the right environment for all our body's own metabolic responses to work effectively.

WHY IS WATER IMPORTANT?

Water plays a vital role in enabling our body to function properly. It is especially important for weight management because it swells food cells and helps our body absorb vital nutrients. Water makes us feel more satisfied with the food we have eaten because it bulks it up, thus stretching the stomach wall and sending messages to the brain telling us we are full. Also, the water content in blood helps the absorption and transportation of all the nutrients, vitamins and minerals in the body and helps flush out all the waste products from the system. When you change to a healthier diet your body will initially produce more toxins and you will need to rid the body of these with water.

So the second step of the Body Blitz Plan is to **drink more water**. In this chapter you'll learn about the effect of different drinks on your body and how to:

- Get out of the habit of drinking too many of the wrong sort of drinks.
- Get into the habit of giving your body the water it needs.

Body Blitz Must Dos:

The three keys to successful hydration are:

1. Drink a minimum of two litres (eight glasses) of water a day, spread evenly throughout the day.
2. No more than two cups of coffee or tea or two cans of fizzy drink a day.
3. No more than ten units of alcohol a week.

ARE YOU DRINKING ENOUGH WATER?

To help you find out what your hydration levels are like, answer the questions in the following quiz.

1. What colour is your urine?
   a. dark yellow
   b. yellow
   c. almost clear

2. When did you last have a drink of water?

    a. more than two hours ago

    b. one to two hours ago

    c. within the last hour

3. How often do you go to the toilet in the day?

    a. less than twice

    b. two to four times

    c. more than four times

4. How many cups of tea/coffee/fizzy drinks do you drink a day?

    a. five plus

    b. two to five

    c. one to two

5. How many glasses of water do you drink a day?

    a. one to four

    b. four to eight

    c. eight to twelve

6. How often do you feel thirsty?

    a. never

    b. sometimes

    c. frequently

7. When you drink alcohol do you drink water as well?

    a. never

    b. sometimes

    c. always

If you answered:

MOSTLY A'S

If you scored mostly A's you are probably unaware of the importance of water. It is likely that you are acutely dehydrated, which means you lack the appropriate amount of water for your body to function properly both when exercising and in everyday life. This is putting a lot of pressure on your system, which in turn will have a direct impact on your energy levels without you even realizing it.

Action: Take action NOW! Cut down your tea and coffee intake to a maximum of two cups a day. Drink a glass of water immediately after exercise and sip water during your exercise session. Start to build up your water intake to two litres a day. Begin by adding two glasses of water to your existing intake and add an extra glass each week until you reach your quota.

MOSTLY B'S

If you scored mostly B's you are aware of the importance of water but you still have a little way to go to bring your body up to its right hydration state. It is likely that your body is in a state where it is never fully hydrated to meet the demands placed on it day in and day out. The water you are drinking should be better spread out during the day to help hydrate your body consistently.

Action: Focus on increasing your water intake to eight glasses a day. Spread these out throughout the day to avoid excess stress on your bladder and the need to rush to the toilet the whole time.

MOSTLY C'S

If your scored mostly C's you are doing a good job of fulfilling your hydration needs. Your body is starting to tell you when you need to drink and replenish your fluids.

Action: Work on increasing your intake of fluids at the start of the day. This will have an immediate effect on your energy levels to set you up for the day. Plan to hit your water intake of eight glasses each day, whatever the circumstances and spread the water intake evenly throughout the day.

How to Check Your Hydration Status

1. Look! Your urine should be a very pale yellow straw colour.
2. Taking vitamin supplements will affect the colour of your urine. To get a true colour reading, pass water twice after taking the supplements before checking the colour of your urine.
3. Check your body weight. Weigh yourself before your **structured exercise** session and establish a baseline weight before exercise. Weigh yourself immediately after your exercise session – every pound lost in weight equals a loss of two cups of fluid. You will then need to replace this loss of fluid by drinking water. Do not fall into the trap of thinking this decrease in weight is a loss of body fat. Unfortunately body fat takes longer than a one hour exercise session to disappear!

THE LOW-DOWN ON HYDRATION

HOW MUCH WATER SHOULD I DRINK?

It is generally agreed that we all need two litres of water a day. This figure is the minimum – if you exercise a lot, travel, have a high fibre diet, live in a hot climate or work in an air conditioned office your water intake should be higher, at least two and a half litres a day. And if you think that's a lot consider the advice professional athletes are given – in hot weather it's eight litres a day!

You can drink either tap water or mineral water, whichever you prefer – drinking too much sparkling mineral water however might cause stomach discomfort.

CAN I DRINK ALL MY FLUID IN ONE GO?

It is much better to space out the fluid you drink throughout the day. Imagine it in this way:

> *Imagine your body as a plant in a flowerpot which has not been watered properly for a few weeks. Its leaves are drooping and it is looking rather sorry for itself. The plant clearly needs water but if we watered it with all of the water it needs in one go, then the water would flow out the bottom of the flowerpot and very little would be retained by the soil to feed the plant. However, if the same amount of water is fed to the plant little by little, allowing the plant to absorb the water, then the plant will hydrate back to its former glory. The same concept applies with the body. If we go too long without consuming the proper amount of fluid and then we consume it all in one go, the bladder and kidneys have to work exceptionally hard and we will just end up making frequent visits to the toilet as most of the water will pass straight through us, rather than being retained as needed in the body.*

WHY DO I RARELY FEEL THIRSTY?

If you rarely feel thirty it is likely that the message centre in your brain that tells you when you are thirsty has become lazy and has lost the ability to give you the right message that you need to drink. Quite simply, your body has got so used to being chronically dehydrated that this is now its normal state. In addition, the hydration message centre is very close to the hunger message centre in the brain, so it is likely that any messages you are receiving will be interpreted as you needing to eat rather than needing to drink. The good news is that you can re-educate or retrain your brain so your thirst mechanism centre starts to tell you to drink again. By gradually increasing your water intake you will find that over a period of as little as three weeks your body will start to tell you when you need to drink water.

When you next feel like eating something, ask yourself the question: Am I hungry or am I thirsty? *Always* drink a glass of water before you start to eat something. As I said at the start of the chapter, water is especially important for weight management as it swells food cells and helps our body absorb vital nutrients.

Did You Know?

New research shows that drinking a cup of coffee just before aerobic exercise can actually improve your workout as the caffeine will boost your body's energy release mechanisms.

DO TEA OR COFFEE COUNT TOWARDS MY DAILY WATER INTAKE?

You may think that cups of tea and coffee boost your daily water intake. Unfortunately this is not the case as they are diuretics and actually encourage your body to get rid of fluid. Even though they are a liquid and do contain water they dehydrate the body rather than effectively providing the cells with the fluid they need.

DOES THIS MEAN I CAN NEVER DRINK TEA AND COFFEE?

No. For many people tea and coffee are an integral part of the day and there is really no need to forgo them completely. But your intake does need to be moderated. The Body Blitz Plan recommends no more than two cups of tea or coffee a day. These two cups do not go towards your quota of two litres of water a day, so you need to make sure you fulfil your water quota as well.

Studies have shown that drinking tea and coffee can have a mild health benefit. For example, a single cup of tea, with or without milk, provides a useful source of flavonoids, which act as antioxidants and can help to protect the body against heart disease and cancer. Green tea, which is very popular in Asia, has the highest concentration of flavonoids. But remember, even though there are health benefits, tea and coffee contain tannin and caffeine, which can inhibit the absorption of the essential nutrients calcium and iron. You should also be aware that if you have a cup of tea or coffee in the morning with a multivitamin tablet, the tannins and caffeine can inhibit the absorption of essential nutrients.

But It's So Bland!

If the taste of water doesn't do anything for you, then you can flavour the water with a twist of lime or lemon or add a splash of freshly squeezed orange juice. Alternatively, you can add a slice of lemon and a chunk of fresh ginger to hot water (this is particularly cleansing first thing in the morning).

Fruit juice cordials can be a great way to make your water intake a little more interesting – but do watch the calorie content. For example, a 250 ml glass of pink grapefruit squash made with one part juice and 4 parts water will give 88 calories. Hit your 2 litre quota of 8 glasses of this, and that is a whopping 704 calories without you even eating anything! Reduced sugar and low calorie cordials can help you keep the calories down while helping to boost your fluid intake but always have a look at the labels for hidden calories that can sneak up on you without you realizing. In addition, some of these cordial drinks can contain a lot of artificial sweeteners, which are not necessarily as healthy for you as natural sugars. So the general rule is, if you need to flavour your water with cordials keep them weak to act as a hint of taste rather than a concentrated flavour burst! Diluted cordials are especially helpful when you need to hydrate your body after exercise.

Herbal teas can be another great way to boost your fluid intake, though not all are stimulant-free. Some herbal teas such as fennel and dandelion are particularly good to drink because they contain properties that can assist in ridding your body of toxins. So drinking herbal teas can contribute towards your two litre target. However, because water really is the gold standard, a good tip to follow is to make five of your eight glasses of fluid a day WATER.

IS IT OKAY TO DRINK ALCOHOL?

For many of us alcohol is a pleasurable part of our lives. But whether we like it or not, alcohol is a major hindrance to long-term fat loss and weight management. This is for two reasons:

1. Alcohol provides a lot of empty calories that have no nutritional value for the body. It provides seven calories per gram, which will significantly increase your total calorie intake if you consume large quantities. In addition, many alcoholic drinks contain sugars and other carbohydrates which increase your calorie intake further.

2. Calories from alcohol, unlike the energy we derive from carbohydrate, protein and fat, cannot be stored by the body. This means that any calories we consume from alcohol have to be burnt off by the body *before* the body can burn off calories from other sources of food – no matter how nutritious these foods might be. Any excess calories that haven't been burnt off during the day, regardless of where they have come from, will simply be stored as fat in the fat cells. Remember, the fat cells have the capacity to keep on getting bigger and bigger!

Watch Out For Those Wines!

Jane was suffering from middle age spread. She had always dieted and generally watched her weight, however as she got older she became extra determined to keep her body fat levels under control. She religiously watched her fat intake and operated a starch curfew but she was overlooking one thing – the amount of wine she was drinking. The two glasses she drank at the end of her day while she unwound before her evening meal soon became a total of five by the end of the evening. By the end of the week this meant Jane was easily consuming an extra 500 calories a day without her really noticing it. Jane says:

'*As soon as I understood how all these calories were adding up from alcohol and how my body was not able to use them, I was able to see where I had been going astray. I have now cut back and I drink more spritzers which help me hydrate at the same time. I have also found that I snack a lot less as I have more willpower to avoid nibbles like cashew nuts and crisps.*'

So how did Jane do? Over the course of ten weeks Jane dropped eight pounds of body fat and she fitted into her favourite skirt, which had been left unworn at the back of her wardrobe for over four years. The extra vitality she felt in the mornings also helped Jane to be more active throughout the day.

SO HOW MUCH ALCOHOL CAN I DRINK?

Doctors recommend that safe drinking levels are between 21 and 28 units per week for men and between 14 and 21 units for women. One unit is a glass of wine, a single measure of spirit or half a pint of normal strength beer.

Some research has shown that moderate drinking – one to two units a day – can actually do you some good as it helps to counteract cardiovascular disease. This works by preventing the blood from clotting, a risk factor leading to heart disease and strokes. However, these benefits only apply to people who are already at risk of heart disease. For women who have not gone through the menopause and men under 40, heavy drinking (more than 10 units at a time) is linked with significantly raised blood pressure.

Because of the calories contained in alcohol the Body Blitz Plan recommends no more than 10 units of alcohol a week. These should be spread out over the course of the week rather than being consumed all in one evening! This would put extra pressure on your kidneys and, more importantly, create a large increase in your daily average intake of calories. Being consistent with your daily calorie and fat gram intake is a crucial factor in your long-term success (see Step Five for more about this).

Some alcoholic drinks contain more calories than others: a single measure of brandy, whisky, gin, rum or vodka contains 50 calories; champagne contains 70 calories per unit; white wine and red wine contain 75 and 90 calories per unit respectively; bottled beer contains 90 calories per unit, and alcopops are the worst offenders with a whopping 215 calories per one to two units!

Alcohol also has a significant dehydrating effect – far more marked than tea and coffee. If you drink alcohol you must ensure you top up your daily water consumption to balance out its effect. If you drink alcohol after exercise in hot weather you will notice the effect of dehydration even more. You'll take frequent visits to the bathroom and lose valuable fluids. More importantly, it will trigger off your thirst mechanism which may act as a stimulus for you to eat more when really it is water you need to be consuming.

Juices and Smoothies

Fruit juices and smoothies can be a quick and easy way to boost your energy levels and hydrate your body. They are also a great way to help you get your five portions of fruit and vegetables a day.

Fruit juices are high in antioxidants, which help to prevent disease and premature ageing. You need to drink fruit juices within two hours of making them for them to be of the most nutritional value. A glass of freshly squeezed orange juice may be as far as you get or you may really get the juicing bug and invest in a juice extractor. Here are some tasty fruit combinations to try – remember to always dilute your juices with a little water to boost your water intake and aid your body's ability to absorb the nutrients:

See the *Body Blitz 14-Day Eating Plan* chapter for more about smoothies.

- asparagus, carrot and cucumber
- kiwi, mango and orange juice
- apple and grape
- apple, carrot, melon and ginger
- tomato, red pepper and cucumber
- carrot, tomato and beetroot
- apple, orange and strawberry
- apple, pineapple and papaya
- apple, asparagus and watercress

Fruit smoothies are also great thirst quenchers and they provide an excellent breakfast on the go or a fantastic energy boost in the middle of the afternoon. They are so tasty you will find your whole family will be wanting one too!

Some commercial smoothies can be high in calories as full-fat yoghurt and milks are often added – so always have a quick look at the label before buying one or ask how they are made if you are in a juice bar.

To add some creaminess to your smoothies without piling on additional calories, pour your favourite low-fat fruit yoghurts into an ice cube tray and freeze. You can then take out the cubes and add them to your smoothie. Alternatively, for speed, you could freeze the whole yoghurt and peel off the container when you are ready to use.

The recipe opposite is a great start to your day:

CREAMY BERRY SMOOTHIE

handful of frozen fruit (I find the bags of frozen fruits of the forest found in the frozen fruit section of your supermarket particularly good)

$1/2$ pint skimmed milk or soya milk

$1/2$ tablespoon wheatgerm

4 cubes frozen fruits of the forest low-fat yoghurt

ice cubes

Put all your ingredients in a blender and liquidize for about 30 seconds. Pour into a glass and drink. Add a little water if you find the consistency too thick. For a change, try frozen mango with frozen peach yoghurt cubes!

Note: You can use either skimmed milk or soya milk in your smoothies. Both skimmed milk and unsweetened organic soya milk provide similar calorie values of 34 and 36 calories per 100ml respectively. Soya milk, as well as being lactose and cholesterol-free, is rich in plant phyto-oestrogens, which have been shown to have a protective effect against some reproductive cancers. So while soya milk may not be everyone's favourite it does have huge health benefits – consuming it in the form of a smoothie where its taste is disguised can be a convenient way to boost your daily phyto-oestrogen intake. If you really can't stand the idea of soya milk try these other good phyto-oestrogen sources: yam, black-eyed peas, liquorice root drunk as tea, kale and dandelion greens!

BODY BLITZ HYDRATION MAKEOVER

Before Sarah started the Body Blitz Plan she was struggling with her weight and lacking in energy. She worked in a busy office where the tea trolley and cafeteria was always on hand. The Body Blitz Plan alerted her to the fact that she needed to address her hydration levels. She started recording her fluid intake over a week noting what she was drinking, how much and when. She could quickly see she was consuming far too much tea and coffee, which she partly did to keep her hunger at bay. At first Sarah thought she would never be able to drink two litres of water a day but with a little bit of effort she was hitting her quota after three weeks. She felt a marked improvement in her energy levels, she felt better able to concentrate at work and her appetite decreased. Even her boss noticed a difference!

Here is Sarah's Body Blitz hydration makeover:

Time of Day	Before	Now
on waking	cup of tea	hot water with slice of lemon
breakfast	cup of tea	cup of coffee or tea glass of water
mid-morning	cup of tea	cup of herbal tea
lunch	can of diet soda	2 glasses of water with meal
mid-afternoon	cup of tea	diluted fruit juice
dinner	2 glasses of wine cappuccino	2 glasses of water glass of wine
total caffeine intake	350mg caffeine	50mg caffeine
total fluid intake	0 litres of water 2 units of alcohol	2 litres of water 1 unit of alcohol

Body Blitz Hydration Tips!

1. Invest in a pull-top drink canister. Fill this up with water and keep it topped up in the car. Sitting in traffic is a great way to keep your fluid levels topped up.

2. When you are in the kitchen have a glass of water on your work surface and drink it as you prepare a meal.

3. Aim to drink a glass of water first thing in the morning and then consume $3/4$ litre by lunchtime. Spreading your water content out over the day avoids putting too much pressure on the bladder.

CHANGING YOUR DRINKING HABITS

Throughout the day there are ways you can change your drinking habits to make sure you drink the right amount of water. We all have different lifestyles and constraints so here are some suggestions that allow everyone to give themselves a tailor-made Body Blitz Plan.

Individual	Lifestyle Constraints	Hydration Solutions
busy mum	tired so you reach for your first cup of coffee for energy boost no time to sit down and drink properly attention more focused on what your kids are eating/drinking rather than what you are eating/drinking tiredness prompts you to drink more tea and coffee grab bottled fruit juices for convenience	• Start your day with a cup of hot water with a slice of lemon. • Drink 2 glasses of water with your breakfast. • Get into the habit of having a glass of water once the kids have gone off to school. • Purchase a pull-top water bottle to have in the car. Make sure it is always full of fresh water. • Have a glass of water as you prepare meals. • Have a glass of diluted reduced sugar cranberry juice or orange juice mid-morning and afternoon. Diluting the juice will increase the hydrating ability of the drink and speed up the energy benefits. • Aim to consume 3/4 of your water intake by 4 p.m. This will minimize your need to go to the toilet during the night. • Go to bed with some water beside your bed.

Individual	Lifestyle Constraints	Hydration Solutions
business woman	easy access to office coffee machine wine at lunchtime working through lunch means you are not eating regularly which stimulates you to grab more caffeine for energy	• Replace mid-morning cup of coffee with herbal or green tea. • Always have a glass of water on your desk. • Take a sip of water before and after making a phone call. • Start serving and requesting water at all meetings • Drink a glass of water with every glass of wine you drink.
experiencing middle age spread	habitual cups of coffee and tea throughout day wine with friends at lunch in the habit of drinking a glass of alcohol as you prepare dinner social drinking occasions with friends and family dependent on coffee and tea as thirst quenchers rather than water	• Drink a glass of water mid-morning and mid-afternoon. • To help you keep track of your water intake have 2 glass jars on your sideboard, one empty and one with 8 small pebbles. Every time you have a glass of water transfer one of the pebbles from the full jar into the empty jar. • Measure out 2 litres of water at the start of the day and aim to have drunk all of it by 9 p.m. • Always pour yourself a glass of water when drinking your daily 2 cups of tea or coffee. • Get out of the habit of drinking tea/coffee every time you complete a task. Replace with herbal tea or water.

Individual	Lifestyle Constraints	Hydration Solutions
girl about town	buy coffee from speciality coffee house on your way to work no time to think about drinking water throughout the day so you often consume all in one go social drinks straight from work	• Start your day with a fruit smoothie to help boost energy and hydration levels straight away. • Purchase a bottle of water on your way to work every morning. Have it on your desk and drink throughout the day. • Purchase a small bottle of water and drink on your way to meeting friends in the evening. • If you have gone out in the evening and drunk a lot of alcohol, consume 2 glasses of water before going to bed.
seasoned dieter	dependent upon coffee as a way of controlling your weight often seek food when you are actually thirsty concerned to drink juices because of their calorie content conditioned to think drinking water will increase water retention	• Drink a glass of water before you eat anything. • Develop the habit of asking yourself every time you want something to eat: Am I hungry or am I really thirsty? • Decrease caffeine intake. • Experiment with fruit smoothies to boost energy levels mid-afternoon and help you hydrate. • Make it a ritual to have a glass of water mid-morning and mid-afternoon. Drinking more water will actually help your body flush out toxins.

Tips from Successful Body Blitzers

Paula:

I endorse Body Blitz's suggestion of leaving a bottle of water by the toilet – that works for me. Every time I go to the toilet it reminds me to drink a glass of water, which I do straight away. That way I hit my quota without even realizing it.

Catherine:

I have two glass jars on my sideboard, one empty and one with eight small pebbles. My aim is to fill the empty jar with the pebbles. Every time I have a glass of water I transfer one of the pebbles from the full jar into the empty jar. It works as a great motivator for me and helps me keep track of exactly how many glasses of water I have actually drunk!

Alexandra:

Drinking loads of water really does stop you feeling the need to binge. What I found very helpful was Body Blitz's suggestion of going out of the kitchen and doing something else if that binge feeling reared its ugly head and/or keeping a jug of water in the fridge plus a whole load of peeled carrots and rice cakes to nibble in emergencies.

A FINAL WORD

So now you have read about the benefits of drinking enough water and seen how you can make small simple changes to your daily routine to make sure your body stays properly hydrated. This is probably the easiest part of the Body Blitz Plan – but it is a key step. Stick to the following action points and you'll be well on the way to a super-hydrated and less hungry body!

Body Blitz Active Action Points:

- Start your day every day with a cup of hot water and lemon.
- Commit yourself to increasing your water intake. Aim to have a glass of water on waking, one glass at breakfast, two glasses mid-morning, one at lunch, two mid-afternoon, and a glass with your evening meal.
- When you feel hungry, get into the habit of asking yourself: 'Am I hungry or am I really thirsty?'
- Always drink a glass of water before eating something.

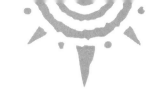

CHAPTER FIVE

Step 3: Figuring Out Fat – The good and the bad

Ask any seasoned dieter what they need to do to lose weight and they'll tell you, 'cut out the fat'. We are right to be aware of the role fat has in helping us address our weight and body fat goals, but focusing solely on the amount of fat we consume does not provide us with the complete picture. It is the total amount of calories we consume in conjunction with the amount of fat and the type of fat that is vital to our success.

The fat in our food is the most concentrated source of energy. One gram of fat provides us with over twice as many calories as one gram of either protein or carbohydrate. Studies show that if we want to lose weight both our calorie intake and the number of calories we consume from fat are important. However, it is important to stress that some fat is important for good health. Certain foods which contain fat supply the fat-soluble vitamins A, D, E, K and some essential fats, which our bodies cannot make for themselves. If we cut out all the fat in our diet we would be depriving our bodies of some very important nutrients.

So the third step of the Body Blitz Plan is to **figure out fats**. In this chapter you'll learn about the role of fat and its impact on the body and how to:

- Cut down on your overall saturated fat intake.
- Increase the essential functional fats in your diet.
- Learn how to read food labels.

Body Blitz Must Dos:

The two key rules to make fat work for you are:

1. Reduce your overall fat intake to around 40 grams a day.
2. Make sure you have at least 15 grams of the right fats in your diet a day.

DO YOU KNOW YOUR FATS?

Answer the questions in the following quiz to help you find out how much fat and which types of fat you are currently eating.

1. Do you always buy reduced-fat products?

   a. yes

   b. no

2. Do you consume three servings of oily fish a week?

   a. yes

   b. no

3. Which of the following cooking methods do you mostly use?

   a. steam, grill, poach

   b. stir-fry, fry, deep-fry

4. Do you eat cheese on most days?

   a. no

   b. yes

5. Do you use olive oil liberally believing it to be healthy?

a. yes

b. no

6. Do you try to cut all fat out of your diet thinking it is the best way to lose weight?

a. no

b. yes

If you answered:

MOSTLY A'S

You are aware of the fat content of foods; however it is likely that you are not getting enough of the right essential fats. In addition, you may perceive that your overall fat intake is low but the quantity of the lower fat versions you are consuming may be large. Alternatively, you may be adding additional calories to your daily intake by consuming excess olive oil. As you will see later in the chapter, even though olive oil is a healthy fat it still provides 47 calories per teaspoon.

Action: Read your food labels and be aware of the amount of olive oil and other oils you are consuming in dressings and stir-frying.

MOSTLY B'S

Your total fat intake is likely to be high due to your intake of visible fats and invisible fats. In addition, it is likely you are consuming a greater proportion of saturated fat, which is associated with an increased risk of heart disease and clogging of the arteries (atherosclerosis).

Action: Cut down your overall intake of fat by reducing the amount of visible fats you are consuming. In addition, aim to consume three servings of oily fish a week.

Visible and Invisible Fats

As we discussed in *The Body Blitz Lifestyle* chapter, visible fats are foods that contain an obvious fat content. The fat we see on meat, as well as foods such as butter, lard, cream and oils are all examples of visible fats.

Invisible fats are foods that do not have an apparent fat content. These fats may make up some of the ingredients in a recipe or they may be found in specific foods with a naturally high fat content that we are often unaware of. Chocolate, avocado, coconut and taramasalata are all examples of foods containing invisible fats.

THE DIFFERENT TYPES OF FAT

All fats provide nine calories per gram, but the different fats perform certain functions in the body and consequently the health qualities of each fat are quite different.

SATURATED FATS

Saturated fats are non-essential fats. As I mentioned earlier, eating too much saturated fat is associated with an increased risk of heart disease and atherosclerosis. These fats do not play a healthy role in the body – in fact, when we consume a diet high in saturated fat the simplest thing for our body to do with it is to transport it to the fat cells and dump it there. Quite simply, the fat cells welcome the saturated fat we eat with open arms and our fat cells get bigger and bigger, our shape gets larger and larger, our clothes get tighter and tighter and our health risks get higher and higher. Butter, lard, cheese and fat on meat are all examples of saturated fat.

TRANS FATS

Trans fats are also non-essential fats as they have no functional health role to play in the body. They are man-made fats produced during hydrogenation of vegetable oil – a process used in the manufacture of various foodstuffs such as margarine. Their consumption is associated with an increased risk of both cancer and heart disease. The majority of trans fats in the diet come from processed foods – look for the word hydrogenated on your food labels and you have found trans fats!

POLYUNSATURATED FATS

Polyunsaturated fats have a very important health role to play in the body, such as helping to decrease blood cholesterol levels. Polyunsaturated fats are divided into two groups – **omega-3 essential fatty acids** and **omega-6 essential fatty acids**. They are considered to be 'essential' because we are unable to manufacture them in the body.

Omega-3 essential fatty acids are found mainly in fish oils as well as flax seeds and pumpkin seeds. Salmon, herring, sardines, trout, pilchards and mackerel are all good sources of omega-3 fats – tuna fish is not such a good source of omega-3 but as a low-fat alternative to meat and cheese it is a healthy option for the family. It is widely believed that omega-3 essential fats help prevent atherosclerosis and help lower blood pressure and triglyceride levels. Omega-3 fats make blood platelets less sticky and less likely to clog, thus decreasing the risk of artery blockage and heart attack. Eating three servings of oily fish a week or using flax seed oil as part of your salad dressing will help you hit your omega-3 fatty acid quota.

Omega-6 essential fatty acids are found mainly in hemp, pumpkin, sunflower, safflower, sesame and corn oil. About half of the oils found in these seeds are from omega-6 fatty acids. Omega-6 fatty acids, like omega-3 fatty acids, have an important function in the body. They are involved in preventing blood clots, lowering blood pressure, helping to maintain the water balance in the body and helping the body to stabilize blood sugar levels.

So as you can see, both of these fats are very important for our bodies. In addition, they actually help us burn protein, carbohydrate and fat. This means that if the fats we eat are from these essential fat sources they will play an important role in the healthy functioning of our bodies before what is left of them is transported to the fat cells and stored.

Cooking With Fats

Be careful when cooking with polyunsaturated fats – they can become damaged when heated at high temperatures, which decreases their health benefits. Monounsaturated fats such as olive oil are a better choice to cook with because they are more stable than polyunsaturated fats.

MONOUNSATURATED FATS

Monounsaturated fats have been coined the most healthy fats, partly because research has shown that the 'Mediterranean diet', with its high olive oil content, can help lower cholesterol levels and prevent heart disease. However, what we fail to remember is that a tablespoon of olive oil will give us the same amount of calories as a tablespoon of melted dripping! So the total amount of fat is still important. Sources of monounsaturated fat include olive oil and rapeseed oil.

So we have established so far, you *do* need to cut down on your overall fat intake, especially your saturated fats, but we have also seen that some fats are good fats and are in fact very important for our health.

ALL ABOUT FATS

Fat Type	Typical Sources	How Do I Spot Them?	Health Effects	Body Blitz Advice
saturated fats (non-essential)	meat, dairy products and some tropical oils including palm oil and cocoa butter	generally solid at room temperature, e.g. butter, cheese, coconut oil	increases cholesterol levels; increases risk of heart disease and certain cancers	The less the better! Should make up no more than 8% of total calories.
trans fats (non-essential)	margarine, shortening, fried foods, breads, crackers, snack foods, spreads, processed/ready-prepared foods	look for the term hydrogenated or partially-hydrogenated fat on food labels – often found in low fat spreads	has a negative effect on cholesterol levels; may increase risk of heart disease and breast cancer	The less the better, minimize consumption. Avoid products that use the words 'hydrogenated' or 'partially-hydrogenated' on the food label.
mono-unsaturated fats (essential)	olive (preferably cold pressed), rapeseed, canola, almond, cashew, hazelnut, macadamia, pecan and peanut oils	generally liquid at room temperature	beneficial effect on cholesterol levels; lowers bad blood fats and increases good blood fats; helps prevent heart disease	Olive oil and rapeseed oil are your best choices. These should make up 12% of total calories.

Fat Type	Typical Sources	How Do I Spot Them?	Health Effects	Body Blitz Advice
poly-unsaturated fats: These are made up of two sub types: **omega-6 essential fatty acids** and **omega-3 essential fatty acids**	vegetable oils and fish and fish oils	generally liquid at room temperature	helps prevent atherosclerois (the furring of the arteries); helps lower blood pressure and cholesterol levels	These are the healthier fats, but should make up no more than 10% of total calories.
omega-6 essential fatty acids	corn, safflower, sesame, soybean and sunflower oils, nuts and wheatgerm	the extracted oils of these foods are liquid	thought to boost the immune system, but watch out as too much vegetable oil can alter the delicate balance of omega-6 and omega-3 fats	Limit consumption of these vegetable oils. Mayonnaise and salad dressings are often made with these – substitute with olive, canola and flax seed oil.
omega-3 essential fatty acids	cold water fish (salmon, mackerel, herring, halibut, tuna and sardines), flax seed, hemp seed, walnuts and their oils, canola and soybean oils, green leafy vegetables	the visible strands of fat on these fish are rich in omega-3 fats	inhibits blood clots; reduces risk of heart disease; increases immune function	Most people will need to increase consumption to reach the ideal 3.6g daily.

Useful Measures:

One teaspoon of oil provides 5 grams of fat and 47 calories.

One tablespoon of oil provides 15 grams of fat and 141 calories.

THE LOW-DOWN ON FAT

WHY DO WE NEED TO EAT FAT?

Although most of us eat far too much fat in our daily diet, we do need some. Here are some reasons why:

- All types of fat give us nine calories per gram so it provides a valuable source of energy.
- It helps the body produce key hormones that regulate various bodily processes.
- It helps transport and absorb carotenoids, a group of powerful antioxidants, and the fat-soluble vitamins A, D, E and K.
- It gives us our shape and a glow of health as opposed to looking gaunt and bony.
- It acts as a thermal blanket keeping us warm and defending the body against heat loss.

HOW MUCH FAT SHOULD WE EAT A DAY?

It is often recommended that fat intake should be no more than 30% of the total calories eaten each day. But percentages can be misleading – 30% of a 5,000 calorie diet is a lot more than 30% of a 1,500 calorie diet. Although percentages can give us a useful rough guideline, the most important thing is to keep track of the total amount of fat grams you are eating in your diet. **The Body Blitz Plan recommends a daily fat intake of 40 grams** and a calorie intake range of between 1,200–1,500, dependent upon your activity levels, diet history and stage on the plan.

The Body Blitz Plan will help you keep track of your fat gram intake. The recipe section is full of foods and meal ideas that will help you stay within your 40 gram fat budget. You can also learn a lot about your total fat intake by reading food labels to check the amount of fat in the product. Some labels will even specify the types of fats.

WILL I STILL LOSE WEIGHT IF I CUT DOWN ON CALORIES BUT NOT FAT?

While you may initially lose weight, if you cut down on your calories but you still have a high fat intake you will experience frustration at not reaching the weight you want to be. This is because you will still have more fat in your diet than your body is able to use and the easiest thing for the body to do is to store it as body fat in the ever-adaptable fat cells. In addition, it is likely that you will feel hungry as the volume of food you consume will actually be quite small due to the fact that fat has such a high calorie value for the amount consumed.

IF I EAT ONLY REDUCED FAT OR LOW-FAT PRODUCTS WILL I LOSE WEIGHT?

While the aim is to keep the total amount of fat down and purchasing reduced fat versions of regular food may seem a convenient way to achieve this, studies have shown that individuals who think they are eating low-fat products actually consume more of them because they think they can thus push up their total calorie intake. So spreading your bread with an extra thick layer of low-fat cream cheese is no different from spreading the same piece of bread with a thin layer of regular fat cream cheese. So if you hate the idea of eating reduced fat versions of regular foods then your strategy should be to eat the normal product but watch the amount you eat.

HIDDEN FAT GRAMS IN EVERYDAY SNACKS

You might be surprised at just how much fat is contained in the fast foods we love to snack on! Some of the snacks listed below will actually use up half a whole day's Body Blitz fat budget in one go…

SNACKS	GRAMS OF FAT PER PORTION
packet of crisps (30g bag)	9
slice of hot buttered toast – butter oozing off!	10
2 cream crackers with a wedge of cheddar cheese	20
slice of pepperoni pizza	10
1 pitta bread with a serving of taramasalata	30
bar of chocolate (50g bar)	15
packet of peanuts (50g packet)	25
1 scone	7
1 bagel	2
1 rice cake	0.5
piece of fruit	trace

Remember, fat grams are not the whole story – total calories are also important (the **starch curfew** will help you here). But the selection of what you nibble on can really impact your daily fat gram budget. But don't despair. For all those fat-filled foods we love to eat, there are plenty of healthier, lower fat alternatives available. Going low-fat certainly doesn't have to mean sacrificing flavour either. Have a look at this range of high-fat foods and their healthier lower fat substitutes.

LOW-FAT ALTERNATIVES TO HIGH-FAT FOODS

FOOD	GRAMS OF FAT PER PORTION
cream	
double cream (1 tablespoon)	14
double cream, half-fat (1 tablespoon)	7
single cream (1 tablespoon)	8
natural bio yoghurt (150g pot)	4
yoghurt – low-fat, plain (150g pot)	0.3
fromage frais – low-fat (1 tablespoon)	0.05
fat-free Greek yoghurt (1 tablespoon)	0
chips	
thin cut (burger bar portion) (125g portion)	22
thick cut (fish and chip shop portion) (250g portion)	35
oven (200g)	7
baked potato, large	0.1
pork chop	
grilled with fat left on (165g)	21
grilled with fat removed (135g)	9

FOOD	GRAMS OF FAT PER PORTION
cod	
fried in batter	9
poached	1
chicken (100g)	
roast meat (light and dark), with skin	14
roast dark meat, no skin	7
roast breast meat, no skin	4
turkey (100g)	
roast breast meat, with skin	6.5
roast breast meat, no skin	1.4
roast dark meat, no skin	4.1
cheese	
cheddar (50g)	17
Edam (50g)	12
low-fat cheddar (50g)	8
cottage cheese (2 tablespoons)	1.5
mini cheese spread triangle	4
milk (one cup)	
whole	8
semi-skimmed	3.2
skimmed	0.2

FOOD	GRAMS OF FAT PER PORTION
spreads (enough to cover one piece of bread but not too thick!)	
butter	8
margarine	8
low-fat spread	3
cream cheese	2.8
reduced fat cream cheese	1.6
quark	0.3
dips (1 heaped tablespoon)	
taramasalata	23
hummus	11
guacamole	8
tzatziki	4
sour cream onion dip	7
mayo (1 heaped teaspoon)	
mayo	12
reduced fat mayo	4.5
breads	
croissant, medium	12
focaccia (75 g)	4
1 crumpet, medium	0.3
1 potato cake, medium	1
1 bagel, large	2
1 pitta	2
slice wholemeal bread	1
slice of ryvita	0.7

BODY BLITZ HEALTHY FATS MAKEOVER

Heather, a busy mum, turned to Body Blitz when her weight loss efforts were not paying dividends. Heather was conscious about her weight but she was also careful not to give the wrong example to her children about weight loss by going on fad diets or being fussy with her food. Consequently, Heather's diet was fairly balanced but she did need to cut down on the amount of fat she was consuming. I encouraged Heather to write down what she ate for a week and quite soon we were able to identify several high-fat culprits that made a regular appearance. Below you will see Heather's revamped healthy fats eating plan.

Meals	Before	Now
Breakfast	2 slices toast with butter and marmalade, cup of coffee	Swiss muesli with live bio yoghurt
Lunch	jacket potato with butter and sweet corn, side salad with mayo	open sardine green salad sandwich (no mayo)
Mid-afternoon snack	50g chocolate bar	creamy berry smoothie (see page 75)
Dinner	lasagne with salad dressing and garlic bread, ice cream	provencale-style poached chicken with vegetables (see page 193), fruit salad

Heather was really pleased with her makeover – not only did she have more energy but she felt really confident that she was giving her children a positive message about healthy eating while she achieved her body fat goals. She particularly enjoyed the creamy berry smoothie which she had while the children had their tea.

So how did she do?

Over twelve weeks Heather lost two inches off her waist and two inches off her belly button measurements and she decreased her body fat by three percent, which brought her body fat into the healthy body fat range for her age.

IN THE KITCHEN

It's not just the individual ingredients and the types of food we eat that make a difference. Different ways of preparing foods can also have a big impact on the final fat gram count of each meal.

Cooking method	Lower-fat alternatives
frying	Bake, steam, grill
stir-frying	Blanch vegetables in boiling water first and then flash stir-fry in seasoning.
stews and casseroles	Brown off the meat first in a small amount of liquid. Or prepare dish a day ahead of serving and skim off fat from top of the dish.
deep-fat frying	Experiment with microwaving and en papillote – a method of cooking in which food is wrapped in greaseproof paper or foil and baked in the oven. Works well with vegetables and seafood. Adding a little liquid such as citrus juices or wine and herbs can help keep food moist as well as adding flavour.
roasting	Can be a no-fat cooking method. Use a metal stand (trivet) to help fat drain away from food. If basting required, try brushing with oil to reduce the quantity used and mix with balsamic and sherry vinegar to make a small amount of oil go further.

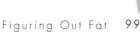

Body Blitz Cooking Tips

- Purchase a good sharp knife to trim all visible fat from food prior to cooking.
- Pour olive oil or flax seed oil into a spray canister and use to spritz salads and lightly grease pans.
- Remove all visible fat from meat before cooking.
- Invest in a good quality non-stick pan.
- Blanch veggies in boiling water prior to stir-frying – this minimizes the fat you will require in the stir-fry pan and the vegetables will retain more of their nutritional value while absorbing minimum fat.

READING FOOD LABELS

If you really want to get your fats sorted you will need to get into the habit of examining food labels. These days all packaged foods are required to carry detailed labels explaining the nutritional value of the product. A typical food label will look something like this:

AVERAGE VALUES	PER 100g	PER 300g PACK
Energy	305kj 70kcal	915kj 210kcal
Protein	6.1g	18.3g
Carbohydrate, of which sugars	9.6g 0.8g	28.8g 2.4g
Fat, of which saturates	1.9g 0.6g	5.7g 1.8g
Fibre	1.2g	3.6g
Sodium	0.25g	0.75g

The amount of energy in a product is shown as kcal and kj. Kcal or kilocalories are the same as calories; kj or kilojoules are simply another way of measuring energy.

Here is how you read a food label:

1. At the top of the label you will see the information is presented in per 100 grams and per serving. I always advise looking at the per serving information because you have to do less arithmetic and this is actually what you will be putting in your mouth!

2. Look at the total amount of calories. In this example, this food will provide 210 calories per serving.

3. Look at the total amount of fat per serving. This product will provide you with 5.7 grams per serving.

4. Look at the amount of saturated fat. This product provides 1.8 grams of saturated fat.

5. Next check out the list of ingredients. Avoid ingredient such as hydrogenated or partially-hydrogenated vegetable oils and trans fats. As a rule of thumb, the higher up the ingredient list these fats appear the more of them there will be in the product.

Verdict: Total calorie content is 210, total fat intake is 5.7 grams of which 1.8 grams are saturated. Remember your total daily fat budget is around 40 grams so this product is a good selection. It is actually an example of a ready-prepared meal – serve it with three portions of vegetables and a dessert of fresh fruit and natural bio-yoghurt and you have yourself a very balanced meal that fulfils your fat gram criteria.

Beware of the Snacks!

Carol juggled a part-time job and two young children. She would take Toby to school and drop Sam off at the crèche before grabbing a large hot chocolate and an almond croissant from her favourite coffee shop on her way to work.

Carol would often work through her lunch break so she could get away early to run a few errands before collecting Sam and Toby at three p.m. To save time she would grab a bag of low-fat crisps and a reduced fat chocolate bar to munch in the car. Preparing the children's tea inevitably meant she grabbed some of their chips and the odd leftover fish finger! Once the kids had finished eating, she would sit down with her partner Paul to enjoy their favourite cheesy bacon pasta bake.

Once Carol knew about the Body Blitz Plan she could see where she had been going wrong. She learnt how to make better choices on the run; how to read food labels effectively so she was no longer misled by 'reduced fat' labels, and how to have more nutritious snacks throughout the day.

Carol made some healthy adjustments to her daily diet: breakfast became a cappucino, a bagel and a bottle of orange juice; for lunch she brought a thermos of soup from home, which she could have at her desk while she finished her work, or a pitta bread with carrot sticks and a small pot of cottage cheese; in the mid-afternoon she had a frozen banana smoothie, which she would make for herself and the boys, and her evening meal became lamb and vegetable hot-pot (see page 185), or lime marinated grilled salmon with salsa (see page 195) was another particular favourite, which she would serve with potatoes for Paul.

How did she do? After 12 weeks Carol had lost 8 pounds of weight and her body fat had dropped from 36% to 32%, which meant she saw a considerable change in her body shape.

WATCH OUT FOR THOSE MISLEADING LABELS!

As well as nutritional facts, food labels tell us about their contents by using terms such as 'low-fat' and 'sugar-free'. While this can be useful you should be aware that labels can be misleading. One food may be described on the label as 'low-fat' but in actual fact this may be a relative term used to describe the high-fat product against the 'lower fat version'. Mayonnaise is a classic example of this – individuals purchase the 'low-fat' version often thinking they are saving themselves lots of fat calories. This however is often a fallacy.

The information on food labels can help you compare the types and amount of fat in specific foods – which is very useful when a flash on the front of a box does not necessarily tell us the whole story. For example, peanut butter labels may read 'cholesterol-free' – this is true but it never had cholesterol in the first place! Be wary not to fall into the trap that cholesterol-free means fat-free. Some cereal manufacturers claim 'no added fat' on muesli or wholesome cereal products, yet the natural grains have been processed with coconut or palm oils, which are high in saturated fat. So the answer is learn to look at the small print on the food labels and not just to rely on the 'LOW-FAT' or 'REDUCED FAT' label flashed on the front of the foods.

A FINAL WORD

Don't worry if you feel you are a real fat-food junkie – with a little effort you can still really enjoy your food and your desire for high-fat foods will decrease. Remember, this is not about cutting out all fat from the diet but rather reducing your overall fat intake, whilst at the same time increasing those good sources of fats. You *can* do this. Good luck!

Body Blitz Active Action Points

- Cut down on your intake of saturated fats and trans fats.
- Assess which is your most common source of saturated fat. For most people this will be cheese. Depending on your personal attitude you may like to think about these courses of action:

  a. cut out all cheese for the next 7 days
  b. reduce consumption or
  c. purchase lower fat versions.

- Start reading your food labels.
- Look to maintain and even increase your consumption of foods high in essential fatty acids such as oily fish. Build up to three servings a week.
- Stop eating crisps and croissants.
- Consume 40 grams of fat a day.
- For health purposes, fat intake should not fall below 10 grams a day.

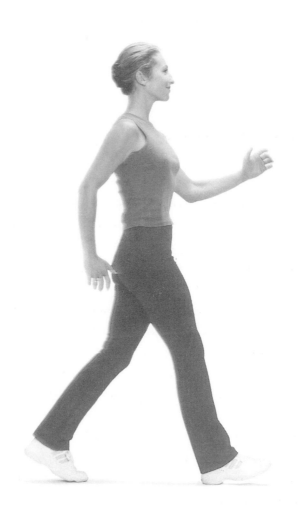

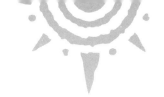

CHAPTER SIX

Step 4: Make Time For Exercise – And say goodbye to fat!

If exercise was a pill – it would be the most widely prescribed medication in the world.

Although it requires a little effort, regular exercise makes you look and feel fantastic. It helps get your body in shape and keeps you healthy both here and now – and for the future too. In fact, it wouldn't be exaggerating to say that exercise is the best investment you can make in life!

These days most people are aware that we have to be active for both our health and successful weight management. Studies have shown that while changing to a healthy diet can be the initial driving force that helps us lose weight, individuals who keep the weight off and body fat down long-term are those who participate in regular exercise and physical activity.

Studies have also shown that although we know we need to take regular physical activity, we often believe that we are getting more exercise than we actually are. Recent studies reveal that we can overestimate our activity levels by up to 40%. We kid ourselves that we're doing enough exercise.

The challenge comes when we try to fit physical activity into our daily lives. So the fourth step of the Body Blitz Plan is to **make time for exercise**. In this chapter you'll learn how to:

- Increase your daily **accumulated physical activity**.
- Start building some sort of **structured exercise** into your weekly routine.
- Establish an exercise plan that works long-term.

Body Blitz Must Dos

1. Fifteen minutes **accumulated physical activity** every day.
2. Three **structured exercise** sessions every week.

WHAT IS ACCUMULATED PHYSICAL ACTIVITY?

This is the energy we can expend in our everyday activities – the sort of activities that you wouldn't describe as 'exercise', such as housework or walking to the bus stop, but which can significantly improve your health and boost the amount of calorie energy you burn up through the week.

This energy will only be burnt however if we physically move our bodies. There is a big difference between being *physically active* and *mentally active* (where our brains are busy all day sorting out problems at work, dealing with families and so on) or *geographically active* (where we move around all day and go to many different locations, for example, picking up the children from school, going to and from work etc., but all the time using every form of transport other than our legwork!)

Accumulated physical activity needs to be done every day. The Body Blitz target is to achieve a daily minimum total of 15 minutes. Whilst the choice of activity is yours, a 'block' of activity should last between 2–15 minutes if it's really going to count. Later on in the chapter you'll find some suggestions for ways you can accumulate activity in your day.

WHAT IS STRUCTURED EXERCISE?

This is your designated exercise session when you will either be exercising at home, in a gym or outside. These sessions typically last a minimum of 30–60 minutes. Later in the chapter you'll learn how to incorporate **structured exercise** into your daily life.

HOW MUCH EXERCISE DO YOU ACTUALLY DO?

Answer the questions in the following quiz to find out just how active you really are:

1. Do you rush around all day using a car, bus or some other form of transport to get you from A to B?

   a. yes
   b. no

2. Does your job demand you sit at your desk all day?

   a. yes
   b. no

3. Do you feel like your 'to do' list is getting longer and longer and you are not achieving anything?

   a. yes
   b. no

4. Do you feel mentally exhausted rather than physically exhausted at the end of each day?

   a. yes
   b. no

5. When did you last get out of breath and break into a sweat?

   a. last week
   b. yesterday

If you have answered:

MOSTLY A'S:

It is likely that you fit a lot into your day but you achieve all your activities by being *geographically active* or *mentally active* rather than *physically active*. Although you are rushing around you are dependent on other forms of transport rather than using your body. This means your total energy expenditure achieved will be greatly reduced.

Action: Complete the **activity audit** to see how you can get more physical activity into your day.

MOSTLY B'S:

It is likely that you are less physically active than you could be. You do get some physical activity into your day but you need to ask yourself where you could physically challenge yourself more.

Action: Start to ask yourself how hard you are actually working when you are physically active. Check out the exertion rate table below to help you. Always aim for a rating of at least four.

EASY EXERCISE OR HARD WORK?

To help you gauge how hard you are actually working when you are physically active, refer to the table below, which I have drawn up so you can measure how much exertion you are putting into your exercise. In **structured exercise** sessions you should be working at an exertion rate of between five and eight. When you are doing **accumulated physical activity** you should be working at an exertion rate of between three and six. As you become fitter, you will find that the exercises you started with that felt like a rating of six will become easier.

To keep your body responding to exercise and expending calories you will need to keep pushing yourself – look at the table below for ideas and aim for activities that increase your exertion rate.

When starting to exercise, do not start out at too hard an intensity – studies show that those who do so quickly drop out of exercise and do not maintain their new found fitness. In addition, if you are new to exercise, it is advisable to check with your GP before commencing your programme.

PHYSICAL ACTIVITY EXERTION RATE

Rating	Exertion	Examples of Exertion	Sweat Factor	Chat Factor
0	none at all	lying completely still in bed, sleeping	no sweat	can chat to your hearts content – if awake!
1	very weak	watching TV at home or film in the cinema, sitting in a meeting at work, sewing, or reading a book	no sweat	can chat to your hearts content
2	weak	browsing in the shops, typing at your laptop, sitting eating dinner, sitting chatting with friends, filling the dishwasher etc.	no sweat	can chat to your hearts content

Rating	Exertion	Examples of Exertion	Sweat Factor	Chat Factor
3	moderate	walking the dog, walking to work, playing leisurely game of doubles tennis	feel a little warm in the clothes you are wearing; starting to sweat	able to talk comfortably
4	quite strong	climbing up escalators, carrying shopping up several flights of stairs, cycling for pleasure	feel like you need to take off an item of clothing; starting to sweat on face and body	able to talk but not sing enthusiastically or loudly!
5	strong: you are physically challenged	manually mowing your lawn, walking very briskly, pushing a pram up a slope, digging in the garden, light jogging	need to take off a layer of clothes to avoid sweating; sweat felt on face and body – you will probably need to pop your clothes into the washing machine once you have finished your physical activity!	able to hold a breathy conversation – but feels a little uncomfortable

Rating	Exertion	Examples of Exertion	Sweat Factor	Chat Factor
6	tough: you feel like you can only carry this on for a limited time	fast jogging or running, carrying and lifting heavy objects such as furniture or weights in a gym	appropriate clothing worn to allow body to breathe; definite sweating on face and body; washing machine necessary for excercise kit	able to hold a sporadic conversation with short pauses for breath
7	very tough: you have to force yourself to do this	running fast to catch the last bus home, skipping with a rope, circuit training	body feeling very warm; sweating; light clothing worn to allow movement	unable to hold a continual conversation – more one word answers
8	very very tough: you are exercising at virtually your flat out pace	running in a competitive race	body feels very hot; sweating felt during and immediately after activity	unable to hold a conversation
9	maximum effort: you can work no harder	running for your life	whole body and head feels very hot	unable to speak

ACCUMULATED PHYSICAL ACTIVITY

BODY BLITZ ACTIVITY AUDIT

As I said at the start of the chapter, there is a big difference between physical activity and mental or geographical activity. Next time you sit down at the end of the day and you feel tired, ask yourself this question: Have I been physically active today or have I just been geographically and/or mentally active? Think about it ...

The purpose of the Body Blitz **activity audit** is to help you check where you can replace geographical and mental activity with physical activity. Write a list of the things you do in your day and where appropriate think about replacing or substituting with physical activity. Depending on your daily activities you may need to do an **activity audit** for each day, or one for your weekly activities and one for your weekend activities. Here are some questions you can ask yourself:

- Where can I accumulate physical activity?
- How do I get around?
- Could I walk faster on my way to the shops?
- Could I walk up the stairs rather than taking the lift?
- Could I walk up the elevator rather than standing still on it?
- Do I overuse my car for all those unnecessary car journeys?

Your list will be unique to you. Once you have completed the **activity audit** you will be able to see more clearly where you can **accumulate physical activity** in your day.

BODY BLITZ ACCUMULATED ACTIVITY MAKEOVER

Let's meet Georgina, a busy executive always rushing around from one meeting to the next – but was she actually being physically active?

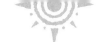

Georgina worked on the seventh floor of a tall office block. She also lived in a flat on the fourth floor. She used the bus and train to get to work but she did walk to and from the bus stop. She did not want to go to the gym and structured exercise did not appeal to her at all. However, she liked the idea of being able to accumulate her activity and by giving her weekly physical activity targets she quickly experienced increased energy and decreased body fat – after three months she even decided to join a gym and start structured exercise sessions.

Once Georgina had completed her Body Blitz **activity audit**, she could clearly see where she could accumulate more physical activity in her day.

Here is her Body Blitz accumulated physical activity makeover:

BEFORE	AFTER
bus to train station	brisk walk to train station
always taking the lift at work	walks up the 7 flights of stairs at work
lunchtime sitting in staff canteen	15 minute brisk lunchtime walk in park en route to collect sandwich
looking after nephew – watching him play in the swimming pool	joins in and swims with him for 20 minutes – even fits in a few lengths for herself while her nephew plays in the 'wet & wild' section of the pool
driving to the supermarket and parking as near as possible to the entrance	parking as far away from entrance as possible to give herself a little extra walk

BEFORE	AFTER
basic walking about the house	now walks briskly up and down the stairs in her flat – as well as walking up the 4 flights of stairs to her flat
pottering around the house – perhaps a spot of hoovering and washing-up	15 minutes vigorous housework i.e. hoovering actively, washing floors etc.
standing on the escalators	walking up the escalators
dropping off her personal post en route in the car	nipping out and posting mail in post box at the end of road
personal assistant fetches sandwich lunch	Georgina now goes herself!

So how did she do?

Within three months Georgina had decreased her body fat from 32.1 % to 28.4%. This represented a decrease of 3.7 % body fat, equivalent to 7 pounds of pure fat. She had more energy, she felt better and she had dropped a clothes size – and this had all been achieved without her once putting on her training shoes and spending hours in the gym. She had accomplished this within her lifestyle constraints of travelling, working long hours and not being a natural keen exerciser.

WHY ACCUMULATING YOUR EXERCISE IS SO IMPORTANT

Think about this…

There are 24 hours in the day, approximately 9 hours of which will be used for sleeping. That leaves 15 hours when we can be physically moving our bodies and expending energy. However, 10 of those hours may be used up at work or with the family where we lead very mentally or geographically exhausting and

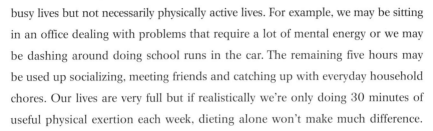

busy lives but not necessarily physically active lives. For example, we may be sitting in an office dealing with problems that require a lot of mental energy or we may be dashing around doing school runs in the car. The remaining five hours may be used up socializing, meeting friends and catching up with everyday household chores. Our lives are very full but if realistically we're only doing 30 minutes of useful physical exertion each week, dieting alone won't make much difference.

Without accumulating our physical activity, when we come to do our **structured exercise** session not only do we need to burn calories in that session to achieve a calorie deficit of 500 calories per day (as discussed in *The Body Blitz Lifestyle* chapter), but we also need to make up for the calories we have not been able to burn throughout the day. This means that we are expecting a lot of results from our one structured exercise session.

So **accumulating physical activity** during the day is an integral strategy not only for long-term successful weight and body fat management but also as an overall improvement to our health. For example, studies have shown conclusively that brisk walking at intermittent times during the day has a protective effect against heart disease, diabetes and high blood cholesterol levels.

STRUCTURED EXERCISE

PLANNING YOUR EXERCISE

Let's be honest, this is the bit that often proves to be the biggest challenge. Getting your head around exercise is sometimes harder than exercise itself!

If you want to get the best out of your exercise plan, there are a few questions you'll need to ask yourself before you start.

- How much weight and body fat do I want to lose?
- How much effort am I prepared to put in?
- How much available time do I have to achieve my goals?

If you have a lot of weight to lose you will need to incorporate both **structured exercise** and **accumulated physical activity** into your Body Blitz Plan. However, if you don't have a great amount to lose and you are not prepared to put in a lot of effort then just watching your nutrition and building accumulated activity may be a more successful strategy for you to stick to long-term. Alternatively, you may find you want to put in the effort but you just don't have the time. In this situation, accumulating your activity and our Body Blitz **Just 10 Minutes!** exercise programme (this is explained later in the chapter) will help you achieve your weight and body fat goals.

GETTING MOTIVATED

There will always be temptations that crop up to throw us off our good intentions of exercising. However remember: to decrease body fat and increase health you do not need to be exercising madly every day – you just need to be a little more active.

To help get yourself on the exercise track, you will need to get a little organized – the following motivation tips should prove useful.

BODY BLITZ MOTIVATION TIPS

- **SCHEDULE:** Plan your exercise sessions at the start of each week and put them in your diary as an appointment. That way that time cannot be allocated to other activities.

- **BE PREPARED:** If working out at a gym, prepare a small shower bag of small bottles of shampoo, conditioner, and moisturizers so all your personal essentials are easily transported to the gym and you don't feel like a carthorse lugging all your kit everywhere.

- **LIMIT TIME:** If new to exercise, plan your exercise sessions to be no longer than 45 minutes – this time is manageable, it will allow you to achieve all you need to, and it won't make you feel you are giving up all your spare time to exercise.

- **REWARD YOURSELF:** Plan a reward at the end of your first six weeks of exercise. Think of this as something that complements your investment in your physical health. For example, you could have a manicure or a massage, or buy yourself some muscle relaxing aromatherapy oils.

- **LEARN TO ARGUE WITH YOURSELF:** Develop the ability to argue with your conscience. Often there may be times when you feel like you don't want to exercise – having the ability to argue with yourself can be a very positive skill to help stop not doing one workout snowballing into a complete break from exercise. Take a look at the following scenario:

The alarm goes off half an hour before your normal rising time so you can get up and do your 20 minute power walk. But instead of getting up you say to yourself: 'I'm really tired so I might as well have the extra 30 minutes in bed'. But your conscience says: 'You made a pact with yourself to do your exercise first thing in the morning.' And your body replies: 'But I'm tired and I really need an extra bit of kip.' Your conscience, however, has the final word: 'Listen! You are going to feel tired anyway and the extra 30 minutes is not going to make all that much difference so you might as well get up and get moving – you will feel better for it and you will not feel guilty for not exercising!'

- **FIND YOUR TRIGGER:** Develop a trigger to exercise. For example, put your trainers by the front door or if exercising first thing in the morning, lay your kit out the night before.

- **FRIEND OR FOE?:** Choose your training partner wisely. Try to workout with a friend who will be able to support you when you feel unmotivated and not encourage you to have a chat and a cappuccino rather than a little sweat. Sometimes friends can be 'exercise saboteurs'!

SO WHAT HAPPENS IN A STRUCTURED EXERCISE SESSION?

As I explained earlier, a **structured exercise** session is a planned exercise time that lasts between 30–60 minutes, and you need to work at an exertion rate of between five and eight. In your **structured exercise** session you should:

- Wear appropriate footwear and comfortable breathable clothing
- Get hot and sweaty
- Get slightly out of breath
- Perform exercises that use the whole of your body such as brisk walking, jogging, bicycling, swimming, aerobic classes, step classes, skipping
- Perform a warm up and cool down (see later in chapter for more about this)
- Be able to hold a breathy conversation – but not a good old gossip with a friend!

Remember to always check with your GP before commencing your Body Blitz structured exercise session.

Structured Exercise Suggestions:
aerobic class
step class
brisk power walk
jogging
running
continual hill walking
cycling
skipping
swimming
stair climbing
dancing
rowing
jumping

VARIETY IS THE SPICE OF LIFE

Once you have incorporated more activity into your daily life and are following a **structured exercise** programme, you will need to add VARIETY to your exercise sessions rather than just exercising for longer amounts of time.

It is advisable to change your exercise programme every 6–8 weeks. This will have major benefits:

- It stops you getting bored
- More importantly for weight loss, it keeps tricking the body so your muscles are continually being challenged to use up calories in different ways!

Here are some suggestions to add variety to your workouts:

- Change the sequence of your exercises
- Change your power walking/running route so you are exercising on different slopes and terrain
- Make one or more sessions a week last a little longer
- Start working at different levels of intensity during your normal workout
- Buy a new home exercise video
- Go to a circuit training class as opposed to your aerobics class.

Good Questions to ask your Gym

If you are doing your structured exercise sessions at a gym, you may find your exercise will be more enjoyable if you know the answers to some of these questions:

1. **When are the busiest times?** Some people may find a busy gym a daunting prospect whilst others may find it is the best way to motivate them. Find out the right times to match your required environment.

2. **How can I keep interested?** Once a month aim to do something new, whether it's a new class, a different teacher or just using a different piece of equipment.

3. **Who are the gym instructors?** Make a commitment to yourself to use your gym instructors – get them to update your programme every six weeks. Not only does this see greatest improvements in your fitness it also keeps you from getting bored.

SO JUST HOW MANY CALORIES AM I BURNING?

Often when we exercise we think we are burning off more calories than we actually are. Consequently, we can lull ourselves into a false sense of security and find ourselves eating more because we think we can. Check out this chart to see how many calories you may typically burn off during some **accumulated physical activities** and **structured exercise** sessions. But remember, exercising is not just about burning calories – it is also about improving your overall health and well-being. When you exercise regularly you will look and feel younger and healthier, and you will have more zest and energy for life.

Activity	Approx. Calories Burnt	Food equivalent
3 mile run	250 calories	50g bar of milk chocolate or 1 small hamburger
1 mile brisk walk	100 calories	low-fat diet yoghurt and kiwi
60 minute step class	350 calories	1 pitta bread with tablespoon of reduced fat hummus
1 hour leisurely cycle ride	200 calories	a medium croissant
food shopping, carrying in food and climbing stairs	50 calories	an apple

Remember: Don't fall into the trap of thinking you can eat a lot more just because you are exercising!

NAVIGATING THE 24

One of the biggest challenges with exercise is trying to find time to do it when you feel your day is crammed full as it is. The way to achieve this is by **navigating the 24**.

As we discussed at the start of the book, to achieve and maintain successful long-term weight and body fat management we need to expend more energy than we are consuming. So if we can burn an extra 3,500 calories over the course of a week – that's a daily burn target of 500 calories – we will lose a pound of fat. This means finding ways to burn an extra 500 calories each day. So how you navigate each 24 hours to achieve these 500 calories is crucial. And to make this effective we need to do it on a regular basis.

There are times when either **accumulated physical activity** or **structured exercise** may be more important to help us navigate our lifestyle challenges. Take a look at the table below to see how we can fit more physical exercise into our busy lives.

HOW TO NAVIGATE THE 24

Individual	Lifestyle Constraints	Exercise Solutions
busy mum	lack of sleep with baby leads to reduced energy levels juggles school runs, part-time job and running a home high domestic stress levels children's meal times always running errands using the car and public transport never seems to be time to exercise high levels of geographical and mental activity leave you shattered	• Try to accumulate 15 minutes physical activity every day. • Schedule in a minimum of one structured exercise session a week and arrange for a friend or relative to look after the children during this time. Try weekends when your partner can look after them – 45 minutes is all you need. • Aim to get your exercise done earlier in the day – that way you have made time for yourself and your body is more receptive to burn fat then.

Individual	Lifestyle Constraints	Exercise Solutions
business woman	entertains with work – eats out a lot high commercial stress levels no time to think about sensible eating and exercise diary always seems full of other activities and meetings meetings running late or rescheduled at last minute encroach on planned structured exercise time got into the habit of using the lift for convenience	● Schedule structured exercise sessions into your diary. ● Complete the 'Just 10 Minutes!' exercises 5 mornings a week. ● Review what form of transport you use to get to and from meetings – can you use your body more? ● Locate stairs in your office building and use them daily!
experiencing middle-age spread	approaching menopause – experiencing weight gain family older and more independent bored never exercised before heavy social calendar with lots of activities with family and friends diary seems to leave no room for exercise always seem to be so busy	● Commit to 3 structured exercise sessions. ● Perform the 'Just 10 Minutes!' mobility and abdominal exercises 5 days a week. ● Complete your activity audit and replace geographical and mental activity with physical activity e.g. brisk walking.

Individual	Lifestyle Constraints	Exercise Solutions
girl about town	socializes a lot breakfast and lunch often grabbed on the run see friends and eat out several times a week always tempted away from the gym to meet up with friends your boss always seems to walk in and want some report just as you planned to go to the gym	• Schedule in your diary 3 structured exercise sessions a week – either at the gym or at weekends outside power walking/jogging with a friend. Do these sessions first thing in the morning – it helps to limit other things getting in the way! • If you are going straight out from work, accumulate your 15 minutes physical activity during the day so you have extra calories burned as a back up!
seasoned dieter	tried every diet around routinely loses and then regains weight – more recently finding it harder to shift the weight and body fat has always thought eating fewer calories is the best way to lose weight, so has never been in the habit of exercising regularly spend a lot of time on your feet so perceive you are more physically active than you really are	• Commit to 3 structured exercise sessions a week. Within 4 weeks you will feel and see the benefits. • Make sure you do 15 minutes of accumulated activity a day. You can achieve this by e.g. walking more briskly and increasing your exertion rating.

EVERYTHING YOU NEED TO KNOW ABOUT EXERCISE

WHAT IS CARDIOVASCULAR EXERCISE?

Cardiovascular exercise or aerobic exercise is any exercise that uses the large muscles of the legs and body. Cardiovascular exercise will involve you getting hot, sweaty and slightly out of breath. Your heart muscle will have to beat faster to meet the oxygen demands of the body to produce energy.

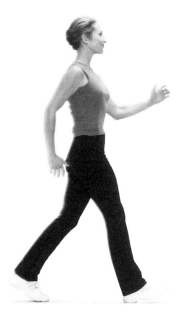

WHAT ARE TONING EXERCISES?

Toning exercises are non-aerobic exercises that are designed to condition and improve the shape of specific body parts. Light weights, body bars, resistance machines and your own body weight can be used to condition and improve the shape of the major muscles of the body.

I AM COMPLETELY NEW TO EXERCISE, WHAT SHOULD I DO?

Being active can take many forms from joining a gym to committing to a walking programme. If you are new to exercise then **brisk walking**, whether outside or on a treadmill, is an excellent way to increase the stamina of your heart and lungs and burn some calories whilst putting minimum stress on your legs – and if done outside it does not cost anything! Here are some helpful hints:

● **First check your footwear** – a pair of supportive walking shoes is a must if you do not own a pair of sports trainers.

- **Aim to build up to walking 20 minutes at a time.** The first time you walk may only be for 5–8 minutes, but by doing it consistently you will soon see an improvement in how far you go and how much more comfortable it feels.
- **Plan your exercise times!** Look at your diary on a weekly basis and plan when you will take your exercise. Make an appointment with yourself and view it as an important meeting that is scheduled regularly. If you miss an 'exercise appointment' look at it in the context of all the positive things you are doing for yourself and do not give up.
- **Your initial target is to exercise three times a week.** However, remember any activity is beneficial and everything goes towards burning calories. Accumulating activity can be very effective at contributing to the total amount of calories your body can burn in a day. Not only is accumulating our activity during the day more convenient for our daily schedule, it has also been shown to have a great impact on our health, specifically reducing blood pressure and blood fats. This is why the Body Blitz Plan encourages you to take regular **structured exercise** sessions *as well as* **accumulated physical activity**.
- **When walking,** aim to walk at a brisk enough pace so that you feel you need to take off an outer layer of clothing. You should be able to hold a brief conversation with someone as you walk. If you find you can hold a monologue conversation, you probably need to push yourself a little harder. Check out the exertion rate chart to give yourself some guidelines.
- **It is a great idea to train with a friend for company** – not only will it make the time go quicker, but you can also motivate each other. However, choose your training partner wisely – try to workout with a friend who will be able to support and encourage you when you feel unmotivated.
- **If walking does not appeal to you,** try your local leisure centre for listings of fitness classes or other sports. Swimming and cycling are particularly good to start with – they are non-weight bearing and place minimum stress on the body.
- **If you are new to exercise,** always check with your GP before starting an exercise programme.

WHEN I START EXERCISING DOES MY FAT TURN TO MUSCLE? AND IF I STOP EXERCISING WILL MY MUSCLE TURN TO FAT?

No. Muscle and fat are very different substances in the body. We have 23 billion fat cells in our body. Even when we lose weight and reduce our body fat we still have the same number of fat cells, but the amount of fat in each cell decreases causing them to get smaller. This is why our clothes feel looser and we go down a clothes size when we lose weight.

Muscle is a protein made up of long fibres that contract creating tension and movement. As we start an exercise programme we may actually increase the amount of muscle or fat-free mass we have in the body. Excess calorie intake, without an increase in the amount of exercise or accumulated activity we do, will make our fat cells get bigger but the muscle fibres will not change into fat cells or vice versa.

I AM REALLY KEEN TO GET A LOT OUT OF MY EXERCISE – SHOULD I DO IT SEVEN DAYS A WEEK?

Exercising is a great way to expend calories. However, it is important to have at least one rest day a week when you do not do any structured exercise.

Having a rest day once a week allows your body to benefit from all the metabolic changes that are occurring in your body as you get fitter and healthier. It will also reduce the risk of injury as too much exercise without rest can cause fatigue in your body.

A good way to look at this is to think how a loaf of bread is baked. The bread has to be kneaded and then left to rest to allow the ingredients to work together to cause the bread to rise. This same concept applies in our bodies when we exercise. Our bodies need to have enough sleep every day and a rest day once a week to allow the metabolic responses to occur that will allow our bodies to get fitter, healthier and leaner.

WHY DO I FEEL MORE SORE 24–48 HOURS AFTER MY WORKOUT?

This is very common when we start a new exercise programme or after a long lay-off from exercise when the body is exposed to unfamiliar exertion. This soreness is generally associated with micro-damage in the muscle, tendons or ligaments. Light aerobic activity such as brisk walking is the best way to reduce the soreness, followed by gentle stretching. If the soreness persists beyond four days after your workout, you may have pushed yourself a little too hard. Remember, it is always better to start gradually and build up your exercise programme. As you get fitter your body will experience less soreness.

SHOULD I EXERCISE WITH A COLD?

If you have a cold, sweating it away could be the worst thing for your body. To help you make the best decision operate what is called the 'neck check':

- If you have symptoms below the neck, (i.e. stiffness, muscle ache) do not exercise – this usually indicates a potential viral infection, which can attack the heart tissue.
- If your symptoms are above your neck (i.e. thick head, runny nose) and you want to exercise then do this with less intensity than usual. If, after starting your exercise session you start to feel worse, stop, listen to your body and wait until you feel better to start again.

Did You Know?

As you incorporate physical activity and structured exercise into your life, you will find it has a carry over effect to other areas of your life. Studies have shown individuals who commence exercise tend to have better dietary habits and eating behaviour, all of which will help towards you reducing your body fat levels.

THE BODY BLITZ EXERCISE PROGRAMME

Now it's time to look at how to put a structured exercise session into practice. Your **structured exercise** session is when you put on your exercise kit and trainers and get a little sweaty! It is a designated time that you have set aside to specifically burn calories and it can last between 30 and 60 minutes.

Whether you are exercising at home, in the park or at a gym, it is always important to warm up before your **structured exercise** session and to cool down after it. We will begin by taking a look at a typical warm up session.

WARMING UP

A warm up is essential before any **structured exercise** because it prepares the body for the work about to be done and reduces the risk of injury. The warm up should consist of some **mobility exercises**, **light aerobic wor**k and **stretches**.

Below is a warm up plan for you to follow before you start your exercise session. Begin with either the mobility exercises or light aerobic activity – and then follow with the stretching exercises. Try to do all the mobility exercises listed but if short of time, at least perform the back exercises (the cat curl and spine rotations). Choose whichever light aerobic activity you prefer – brisk walking or jogging are both recommended. Then finish your warm up with the stretching exercises – for the calves, the hamstrings, the lower spine and quads. Your warm up session should last approximately 10 minutes. *Note:* All the warm up and cool down exercises listed below are described fully later in the chapter.

WARMING-UP SESSION

After the warm-up you can then increase the intensity of your exercise efforts – you may try power-walking, cycling, jogging or swimming. All of these activities, together with the ideas we have discussed throughout this chapter, will help you get the most out of your available time. Remember, the main part of your workout should be between 15 and 40 minutes.

Type of Exercise	Exercise Examples	Purpose	Body Blitz Tip	Time Needed
mobility exercises	side bends, shoulder rolls, spine rotations, cat curl	lubricates the joints preventing them from feeling 'stiff' during the workout. Guards against muscle, tendon and ligament strains	always start with a posture check	2 minutes
light aerobic activity	brisk walking/light jogging	increases body temperature; heart rate increases to increase the efficiency of oxygen transport to the working muscles	by the end of the warm up you should feel like you are warm enough to need to take off a layer of outer clothing. Gradually increase the intensity of your aerobic warm up as you get fitter	minimum 5 minutes
stretching	calves, hamstrings, lying spine stretch, quads	when performed with mobility exercises, helps to guard against muscle, tendon and ligament strain	perform stretches towards end of warm up, once muscles are warm. Hold each stretch position for about 10–15 seconds.	1–2 minutes

If you are short of time, limit your **structured exercise** session to 20 minutes. In this case, your warm up should last for approximately five minutes before you move quickly into the main part of your workout. For your cool down, in the last three minutes of your workout decrease the intensity of your chosen exercise and finish off your workout with some stretching exercises (see below) – the calves, prone hamstrings, lower spine and quads are particularly important.

COOLING DOWN

After you have finished the main workout section of your **structured exercise** session you will need to cool down. The cool down is just as important as the warm up. Stopping your vigorous exercise activity suddenly will cause the blood to pool in the legs. This can cause feelings of light-headedness as well as making it harder for the body to get rid of waste products produced during your exercise. The cool down should consist of **light aerobic activity** followed by **stretching**. Try to do all the stretching exercises listed below but if you are short of time make sure you stretch your calves, hamstrings, lower spine and quads.

COOL DOWN SESSION

Type of Exercise	Exercise Examples	Purpose	Body Blitz Tip	Time Needed
light aerobic activity	light jogging, walking at moderate pace	gradually lowers the heart rate and cools the body temperature; helps to prevent dizziness caused by stopping suddenly; assists the removal of waste products such as lactic acid from the exercising muscles	use whole body movements and gradually reduce the intensity. You may wish to put on a layer of clothing here to reduce large fluctuations in body temperature	2–5 minutes dependent on fitness level. The fitter you are the more efficient your body will become at cooling down
stretching	prone hamstrings, lying spine stretch, quads, full body stretch, neck stretches	lengthens the muscles that have been working; helps to reduce stiffness in the muscles	stretch positions can now be held up to 30 seconds, as the muscle temperature is much warmer. If particularly stiff repeat the stretch positions up to 5 times	time needed 2–5 minutes

What Should I Wear?

Choose clothing that is comfortable during the activity, allows the skin to breathe, and carries sweat away from the surface of the skin. Layer clothing to provide good insulation. A lot of heat can be lost through the head, so consider some sort of head covering. To prevent frostbite in cold weather, invest in a pair of running gloves that allow your hands to breathe whilst reducing heat loss.

JUST 10 MINUTES!

As I mentioned earlier, time is not always on our side when it comes to exercise. The Body Blitz exercise plan however gives you the flexibility to fit different types of fat burning activity into your week depending upon your lifestyle constraints. If you are really short of time though you can always use the Body Blitz **Just 10 Minutes!** programme. This is a great way to help you achieve damage limitation (see Step Five for more about this) when you know you are not going to be able to get to do your normal **structured exercise** session.

Investing 10 minutes of your time to exercise each day will make a big difference to your energy levels, your agility and how you feel about yourself during the day – as well as helping you burn excess calories. So start today – aim to complete first thing in the morning either the **posture** and **mobility exercises** or the **abdominal exercises** (see below) – that way you've done yourself a huge favour even before your day has started! Remember, every small action you take goes towards achieving your weight and body fat goals!

Note: All the exercises listed below are described step-by-step later in the chapter.

Just 10 minutes...
to Better Posture and Mobility

Perform the following posture and mobility exercises first thing in the morning – it will only take you 10 minutes:

1. First do a **posture assessment** – before doing your exercise session you need to make sure you are standing correctly.
2. Now you are ready to perform the **shoulder rolls** – do eight rolls forward and eight rolls backwards.
3. Next perform the **side bends** – four to the right and four to the left.
4. Now take a seat either on a chair or on the side of the bed, keep your feet flat on the floor directly under your knees – perform four controlled **spine rotations** each side.
5. Next come onto all fours and perform your **cat curls** – slowly move through the position eight times.
6. Now lie down on the floor face up and perform the **lying spine stretches** – two stretches on each side of the body.
7. Still lying flat on the floor face up, now perform the **prone hamstring stretch** – move gently into this position and do not stretch too far as your muscles will not be warm and pliable. Hold for 30 seconds for each leg.
8. Now perform the **full body stretch** – hold for 30 seconds and really feel your body lengthen as you do it.
9. To finish, gently come into a standing position and do another **posture check** – preferably looking in a mirror.

Just 10 minutes...
to Flatter Abdominals

Here is a ten minute exercise routine for your abdominal muscles for you to perform first thing in the morning.

1. First perform a standing **posture assessment**.
2. Now lie on the floor on your back and check your posture ready for your **abdominal curls** – perform 12 curls and gradually work up to 30 good quality curls. Ideally, aim to perform the movement slowly and in a controlled manner 2 seconds up and 2 seconds down. At first your curls may take you longer as you focus on performing the movement with good technique and not pulling on your neck.
3. Still on your back, now perform the **oblique curls** – 10 curls to one side and 10 to the other. Again, always perform with good technique and don't rush them – faster does not necessarily mean better! Aim to build up to 30 curls each side.
4. Now come onto all fours and check your posture – your back needs to be as flat as possible. Now you are ready for the **opposite arm and leg reach** – perform 10 reaches each side – ideally 2 seconds reaching out and 2 seconds lowering down. As you get stronger, hold still for 2 seconds the extended position with the arm and leg before lowering.
5. Now finish with a **full body stretch** – hold for 30 seconds feeling the abdominals stretch along the length of the body.
6. Finally, come into a standing position and **check your posture**.

HOW TO DO THE BODY BLITZ EXERCISES

Here are step by step explanations of how to do the exercises that we have discussed in the **warm up** and **cool down** sessions as well as the **Just 10 Minutes!** exercise programme. You can also mix and match the mobility and abdominal exercises below to make up your own **Just 10 Minutes!** programme. Remember it is a good idea to bring variety to your exercise sessions – this will not only stop you from getting bored but it will also keep tricking the body so your muscles are continually being challenged to use up calories in different ways.

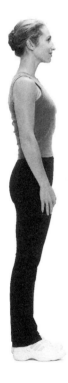

POSTURE ASSESSMENT

The first thing you need to do before you begin your exercise session is to check your posture. This will only take a second and soon it will become second nature.

Good posture is essential to get the most out of your exercise and physical activity.

HERE'S WHAT YOU DO

Stand with your feet hip distance apart with your weight evenly distributed. Soften your knees as you pull up through your legs. Keep the hips square and level. Lengthen through the spine and contract the abdominals, sucking the belly button into the back of the spine as you extend tall. Drop the rib cage, pulling the lower ribs towards the pubic bone. The shoulders should be down and relaxed, so the neck is as long as possible. Breathe smoothly.

AM I STANDING WITH GOOD POSTURE?

To find out how good your basic posture really is, try these simple posture checks. As this is a 'test' there's no need to make extra effort to stand up straight! Just stand normally.

Hand-hip test – it's best to do this with the help of a full length mirror.

1. Standing up, place the palms of your hands on your hips, with your fingers together pointing towards your middle.

2. Standing sideways on, look in the mirror and take note of how your fingers are positioned.

3. If your fingers are tilting forward or backward, your hips aren't in the best position. It's likely your posture can be improved as our hips have a tendency to tilt too far backward or forward.

4. For good posture, your fingers should be close together and pointing down.

5. To correct your posture, try using your abdominal muscles to pull your hips in and up until your fingers are vertical, as in the picture below.

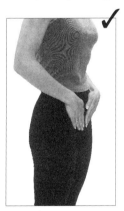 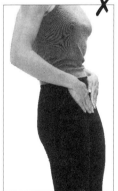 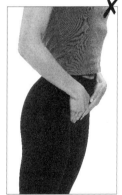

Neck-thumb test – again it's best to do this with the help of a mirror.

1. Stand with your thumbs resting on your collar bones and your palms turned in toward your neck. Spread out your fingers so your little finger just touches your earlobe.

2. Is your little finger vertically on top of your thumb? Or is your little finger further back or further forward than your thumb?

3. For good posture, the little finger should be stacked vertically on top of your thumb, indicating that your head isn't tilting too far forward or backward and putting stress on your neck and shoulders.

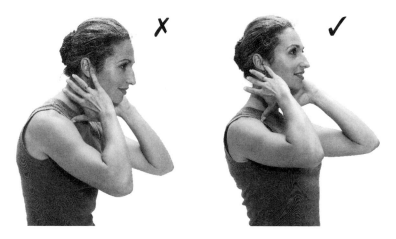

MOBILITY EXERCISES

SHOULDER ROLLS

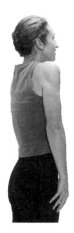

What it does: Mobilizes the shoulder joints and relieves tension on shoulder and neck area.

What you do: First stand with good posture. Then gently roll the shoulders forward, keeping the head lifted and the neck long as you move. Perform eight rolls in one direction and then reverse and perform rolls the other way. Remember to contract the abdominals throughout.

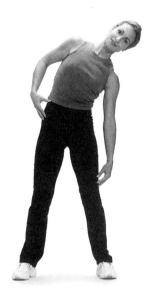

SIDE BENDS

What it does: Mobilizes the lower spine.

What you do: Stand with your feet hip distance apart, with your weight even between both feet. Bend your knees slightly to reduce the pressure on your spine. With your abdominals contracted and your spine long, gently slide your hand down the side of your leg to feel a stretch on your waist. To avoid leaning forward imagine you are going down between two panes of glass, one in front of you and one behind. Keep your shoulders back and over your hips. Keep the lower body still. Repeat in a controlled manner eight times each side.

SEATED SPINE ROTATION

What it does: Releases tension in the middle back.

What you do: Sit up tall on a chair or on the side of your bed. Your feet need to be flat on the floor and directly under your knees. Place your right hand on the outside of your left thigh and reach back with your left hand. Be tall as you turn. You can use your hands as levers to increase the stretch you feel. Only stretch to a comfortable position, holding for 10–15 seconds. Do four spine rotations and then repeat on the other side.

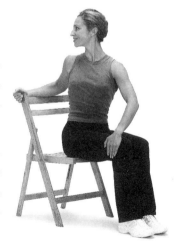

CAT CURL

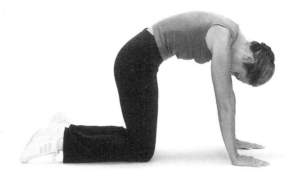

What it does: An excellent stretch for mobilizing the spine.

What you do: Get onto all fours, with your wrists under your shoulders and your knees directly under your hips. Contract your abdominals to arch the back up to the ceiling like a witch's cat. Pay particular attention to the lumbar (lower) region of the back and try to get as much stretch through this area as possible. Contract the abdominals and come back to a flat back position. Imagine you could put a tray of drinks on your back. Next in a controlled manner, let the lumbar spine drop to the floor and let your tailbone point to the ceiling. Repeat the movements up to eight times.

ABDOMINAL EXERCISES

ABDOMINAL CURL

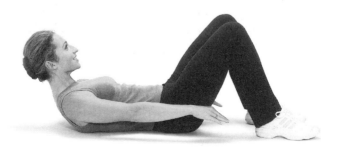

What it does: Tones and flattens the abdominals.

What you do: Lie on your back, the knees bent and feet flat on the floor. Before you start you need to find your neutral pelvis position. To do this, place the heel of the hand on the hipbones and extend your fingertips towards your pubic bone. Your pelvis should be level with the hips neither rolled out to cause the lower back to arch off the floor nor rolled in to create a pelvic tilt. Now place your hands either side of the head – or if you find this too difficult, on the thighs – curl up along the spine. Lead from the breastbone and pull the belly button flat to the floor as you lift and lower in a controlled manner. Ideally aim to perform the movement slowly two seconds up and two seconds down. Breathe smoothly

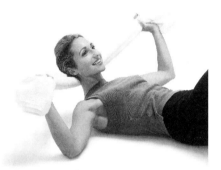

while you perform the exercise and aim to build up to 30 good quality curls each session within three weeks. Technique is very important – but you do need to feel like the abdominals are fatigued when you do this exercise. If you suffer from neck discomfort you can use a towel for support.

OBLIQUE CURLS

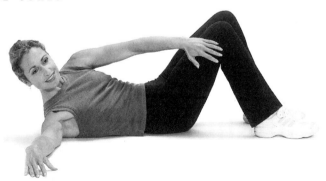

What it does: Targets the waist muscles.

What you do: Lie on your back, the knees bent and feet flat on the floor.

Establish your neutral pelvis position as you did with the abdominal curls. Tighten the abdominals to keep the pelvis fixed and the legs still. Now reach one hand to opposite calf, for example, your right hand to your left calf. As you reach, visualize the belly button being pulled down to the base of the spine. This will avoid the abdominals 'popping' out as you rotate. And think about bringing your bottom rib across to the opposite hipbone. Repeat to the other side. Keep movements slow and controlled. Breathe smoothly and aim to build up to 30 good quality curls each session within three weeks. You do need to feel like the abdominals are fatigued when you do this exercise.

OPPOSITE ARM AND LEG REACH

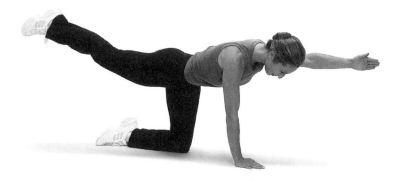

What it does: Strengthens and tones the back and abdominal muscles.

What you do: Get onto all fours with your knees under your hips and your wrists directly under your shoulders. Make sure your back is as flat as possible and strongly contract the abdominals to support the spine and create good balance. Slowly reach forward with one arm and at the same time reach back with the opposite leg. Pulling in your abdominal muscles will help you keep your balance and the flattened abdominal area will help support your body. Slowly bring your leg and arm back to the floor and repeat on the other side. Repeat 10 times each side.

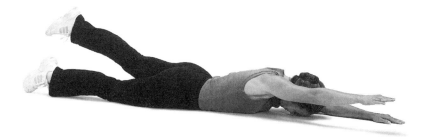

Version Two: If you are new to this exercise or you feel unsteady supporting your weight on one hand and one leg, perform the same leg and arm reaches lying flat face down on the floor with your arms stretched out over your head and the palms of your hands facing down. Raise your arms and legs slightly off the floor as you reach and make sure you are looking down at the floor. As you get stronger progress on to the all fours position.

STRETCHING EXERCISES

LYING SPINE STRETCH

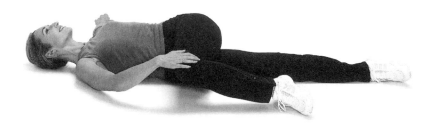

What it does: Releases tension in the lower spine, especially important if you sit at a desk or spend a lot of time in a car.

What you do: Lie on the floor face up with your legs extended flat on the floor. Lift one knee towards the chest and gently ease it across to the opposite side of your body, supporting the outer thigh above the knee with the opposite hand. As far as possible keep the knee at 90 degrees to the torso. You are aiming to get the inside of the knee to the other side of the floor. Breathe in a controlled manner and only do what is comfortable for you. To change sides, contract abdominals and release leg to the floor. Repeat with the other leg. Aim to do at least three stretches each side.

HAMSTRING STRETCH

What it does: Stretches the muscle at the back of the thigh. This is a particularly good exercise to do as part of your warm up.

What you do: First stand with good posture. Place one foot forward with the whole foot flat on the floor. Pull up tall from the spine and contract the abdominals as you gently lean forward from the hips. The supporting leg needs to be bent at the knee. Lifting up your tailbone at the back will increase the stretch you feel on the back of the thigh. Hold for 10 seconds and repeat exercise on the other leg. Make sure you contract your abdominals as you come out of the position.

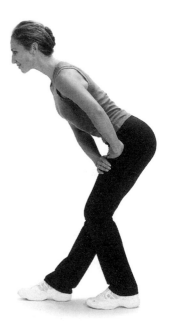

PRONE HAMSTRING STRETCH

What it does: Stretches the muscle at the back of the thigh. This is a particularly good exercise to perform as part of your cool down.

What you do: Lie on the floor face up with the legs bent so the feet are flat on the floor. Gently lift the thigh to the chest and support the leg behind the knee and thigh. Slowly extend the leg straightening at the knee. This will increase the stretch felt on the back of the thigh. Keep the hips flat on the floor and only stretch to a point of feeling a mild stretch on the thigh. Hold for up to 30 seconds. Repeat exercise on other leg.

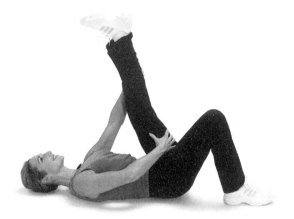

You can use a towel around the foot to help you get a better stretch and feel more relaxed in the upper body.

CALF STRETCH

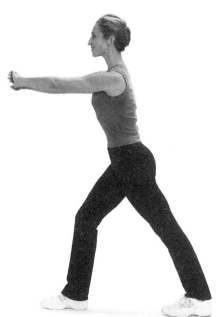

What it does: Lengthens the calf muscles and helps to reduce stiffness.

What you do: First stand with good posture and take a large step back with one leg, placing the whole foot on the ground. Your stance should be about hip distance apart to help with balance and both toes should be facing directly forward. Do check that the toes on the back foot are not pointing out away from the body. Bend the front knee slightly keeping the knee over the ankle – you should be able to see your laces. Press the heel of the back leg into the floor and feel the stretch of the calf muscle on the back of the leg. Hold for 10 seconds. Repeat exercise on the other leg.

QUAD STRETCH

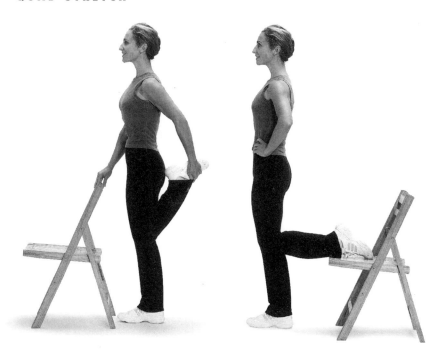

What it does: Stretches the muscle at the front of the thigh.

What you do: Hold onto a chair for balance. Stand with good posture and lift and bend one leg up behind you. Hold onto your shoe laces or ankle with your hand. Keep the knees together and make sure you have a slight bend at the knee on the leg you are standing on. Push your hips forward as the knees stay together. Make sure you keep your abdominal muscles contracted to help you stand tall and avoid arching the back. Hold for 10 seconds and repeat on the other leg.

If you find it hard to support the leg in your hand you can use a chair to rest your foot on.

NECK STRETCH

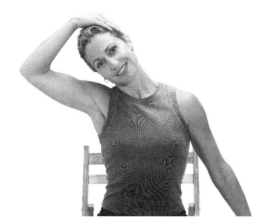

What it does: Stretches the muscles of the neck and relieves tension in the neck, shoulder and upper back area.

What you do: Stand with good posture with your shoulders level and hands down by your sides. Looking straight ahead, gently lower your right ear towards your right shoulder. Make sure your shoulders are still level and gently place your right hand on the upper part of your head in line with your right ear. At the same time stretch your left arm down the side of the body as this will gently increase the stretch you feel on the side of your neck. Hold for 10 seconds. Always move gently in and out of position – depending on how much tension you have may affect the amount of stretch you feel. Repeat the exercise on the other side.

FULL BODY STRETCH

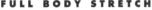
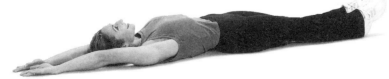

What it does: Stretches the whole of the body especially the abdominal and spine area.

What you do: Lie on the floor face up. Extend your arms above your head. Gently stretch and lengthen through the whole body from your fingertips to your toes. Your lower back may come gently off the floor. Breathe gently and hold for up to 30 seconds. Slowly bring your arms down by your side.

A FINAL WORD

As I said at the beginning of the chapter, exercise is an investment that none of us can afford not to make. There may be times when you really don't feel like it, and sometimes it's okay to listen to your body and not do your **structured exercise** session. But remember, it is the combination of your **accumulated physical activity** and your **structured exercise** sessions that will help you feel healthier and more energetic. You will not only realize your weight and body fat goals but you will also keep in your healthy body fat range. The most important thing is to do something active that you enjoy, then you can be the best that you can be and still live the life you wish to live.

Body Blitz Active Action Points:
- Complete your activity audit so you can work out ways to achieve fifteen minutes accumulated physical activity in your day.
- Plan your structured exercise sessions. If you cannot fit in three a week, place more emphasis on your accumulated activity.
- Have a contingency plan to help you boost your accumulated physical activity levels when you are unable to get to your structured exercise sessions.

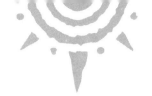

CHAPTER SEVEN

Step 5: Be Consistent – You only have to be 'good' 80% of the time!

How many times have you gone to bed on a Sunday night resolving to yourself that you will be really strict with yourself this week – you will say no to chocolate, sweets or naughty nibbles and you will go to the gym *every* morning before work? And how many times have you actually managed to achieve this? Of course this sort of do or die strategy never works. Even a handful of chips or a mouthful of chocolate will make us feel like we have failed. Such an extreme approach to exercise and dieting just sets us up to feel guilty and frustrated that we are unable to achieve our weight loss goals.

The good news is this: the best way to lose weight, body fat and to stay healthy is not to deprive yourself of everything you love but instead to stick to the **80–20 rule**. With the **80–20 rule**, the key to successful long-term weight loss is consistency rather than being 'good' 100% of the time. If you can stick to the Body Blitz Plan for just 80% of the time you have succeeded! Yes it is true, being consistent means that you can actually eat a little more, you will feel more energetic, you will get the results you are seeking and the best bit is you stop setting yourself up for guilt and 'failure'!

So the final step of the Body Blitz Plan is to **be consistent**. In this chapter you'll learn why consistency is the key to successful long-term weight management and how to:

- Make the **80–20 rule** work for you.
- Develop **damage limitation** strategies that put you in control.

Body Blitz Must Dos:

The three keys to successful weight management are:

1. Stay within a sensible range of calorie and fat gram intake.

2. Work out ways to top up your physical activity.

3. Get to know the triggers that prompt you to eat unwisely.

HOW CONSISTENT ARE YOU?

Answer the questions in the following quiz to find out if you are prone to big swings in your food intake.

1. Do you overeat one day and then under eat the next in an attempt to save your calories?

   a. yes

   b. no

2. If you have binged one day, do you starve yourself the next?

   a. yes

   b. no

3. Do you have a history of dieting?

   a. yes

   b. no

4. Do you go on extreme low calorie diets and then go back to your 'normal' eating habits once you have lost some weight?

   a. yes

   b. no

5. Do you experience plateauing with your weight?

   a. yes

   b. no

6. Do you starve yourself to get into your favourite outfit for a special occasion?

   a. yes

   b. no

7. Do you beat yourself up and think you have 'blown' your diet by having a chocolate biscuit or packet of crisps?

   a. yes

   b. no

8. If you miss a week of exercise do you worry that you have lost all your fitness and next time you won't be able to keep up?

   a. yes

   b. no

If you answered:

MOSTLY A'S:

You are a classic erratic dieter. There are probably large variations in your calorie intake and you find it hard to stick to a fitness plan for long. You are likely to experience great fluctuations in your weight and body fat. In addition, you are probably prone to putting on weight very quickly, especially around times of excess such as Christmas and holidays. Psychologically, you may experience frustration at eating a low calorie diet yet never being able to achieve your weight and body fat goals. You may also feel you are sometimes in a situation of free-fall with your weight, where whatever you try just keeps the scales moving up and not down. You probably also experience fluctuations in energy as you strive to keep your calorie content low one day only to find yourself completely devoid of energy the next and consequently needing to eat more.

Action: Focus first on achieving a **starch curfew** and decreasing your overall fat intake. These two simple steps will automatically help you to be more consistent in other areas.

MOSTLY B'S:

You are probably a fairly consistent eater who keeps their calorie and fat gram intake relatively stable. If you are still having trouble reaching your weight and body fat goals, you may need to have a close look at your diet and exercise strategies to figure out which aspects of your lifestyle are coming between you and your goals.

Action: Put the **damage limitation** strategies into practice (see end of chapter for more about this). Identify what triggers you to eat unwisely, use **portion control** and the **starch-free zone** and increase your physical activity.

DOES THIS STORY SOUND FAMILIAR?

Sue starts her week with great intentions: she eats very little on Monday – no breakfast, a coffee and a diet biscuit for lunch, and a low calorie ready-prepared meal for dinner. Sunday was a dieter's nightmare, she thinks, so she had better make up for all those extra calories she has eaten. She gets through Tuesday with the same determination, although she develops a bad headache from all the coffee she has been drinking to help her concentrate and curb her appetite. Wednesday comes and by 3 p.m. it's no good – the old vending machine calls and two bars of chocolate, a bag of crisps and a Danish pastry pass Sue's lips as hunger and lack of energy drive her to that instant sugar fix. In the evening she feels like she has blown her diet so she grabs some fish and chips on her way home from a few drinks after work. Thursday arrives and Sue still really wants to get into that new outfit she bought for the party on Friday night, so she says no to breakfast (better make up for the fish and chips she thinks), she grabs a slim shake at lunch and a low calorie can of soup for dinner. Friday comes so it's the obligatory no breakfast, can of low calorie soup for lunch and then off to the party. Well, she gets into the dress but she does not feel great, her energy levels are flagging and she feels quite nauseous from eating so little – the first glass of wine hits her very empty stomach … Sue starts Saturday feeling a little bit delicate so masses of toast and butter all round, lunch with friends, drinks in the evening, followed by the cinema with a box of chocolates! Sunday – well, tomorrow is Monday so she might as well enjoy herself today, ready for her 'diet' onslaught again. But this week she vows to be better.

THE VERDICT

If you actually counted out the amount of calories Sue consumed each day, you can see that even though her average daily calorie intake may be in the region of 1,500 calories – which is considered to be 'acceptable' for weight loss purposes – her daily calorie intake has varied from 800 calories to in excess of 3,200 calories. This means that even though she may have consumed on average the right number of calories over the course of the week, she experienced great swings in energy, which culminated in her grabbing the quick sugar fix and not achieving an effective sensible weight loss. The weight Sue will have lost will have been from a loss of water and not a decrease in the size of her fat cells. Also, more importantly, Sue's actions are setting her up for long-term weight loss failure. She will continually feel frustrated as she is depriving herself of food and important nutrients yet never making progress with her weight and body fat goals.

Sue needs to be more consistent – the best bit about being consistent is that it means she can actually eat a little more, feel more energetic, stop beating herself up and get the results she wants.

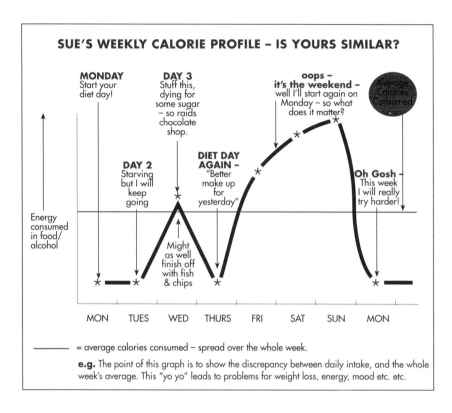

SUE'S WEEKLY CALORIE PROFILE – IS YOURS SIMILAR?

MONDAY
Start your diet day!

DAY 2
Starving but I will keep going

DAY 3
Stuff this, dying for some sugar – so raids chocolate shop.

DIET DAY AGAIN –
"Better make up for yesterday"

oops –
it's the weekend – well I'll start again on Monday – so what does it matter?

Average Calories Consumed

Energy consumed in food/alcohol

Might as well finish off with fish & chips

Oh Gosh – This week I will really try harder!

MON   TUES   WED   THURS   FRI   SAT   SUN   MON

—————— = average calories consumed – spread over the whole week.

e.g. The point of this graph is to show the discrepancy between daily intake, and the whole week's average. This "yo yo" leads to problems for weight loss, energy, mood etc. etc.

THE 80–20 RULE

So as we have already established, the key to successful long-term weight and body fat loss is to apply the **80–20 rule**. With the **80–20 rule** you don't have to be 'good' 100% of the time – you just need to be consistent and stick to the Body Blitz Plan for 80% of the time and you will succeed!

HOW DOES THE 80–20 RULE APPLY TO DIET?

Ideally you will keep your calorie and fat gram content down within a certain daily range. The calorie range for losing weight is between 1,200–1,500 calories per day depending upon how active you are. Applying the **80–20 rule** means you have a 500 calorie cushion each day. As you are also looking at the amount of fat grams in your diet, try and keep these within a range of 30–50 grams a day. If you consistently keep within these bands you will not only lose weight and body fat but more importantly for your health and happiness, you will keep the weight and body fat off. The longer you give your body the opportunity to burn the same range of calories and fat grams the more efficient it will become at using the calories from your food. Applying the **80–20 rule** means that not only will you have more energy but also when you do overeat, your body will be able to use the extra calories more effectively rather than storing them in the fat cells.

Body Blitz Tip

Aim to consume 3/5th of your food by 5 p.m. – this will fuel you with energy during the day and help prevent you overeating in the evening when you are tired and your willpower is at its lowest.

HOW DOES THE 80–20 RULE APPLY TO EXERCISE?

Ideally you should be doing three **structured exercise** sessions a week and **accumulating physical activity** on a daily basis. The **80–20 rule** however allows you to have a more relaxed approach to fitness just so long as you are consistent. There will always be times when you can't get to the gym – and maybe a whole week will go by when you haven't managed to fit in a **structured exercise** session – but there's no need to feel as if you have failed. Remember, how much you weigh in seven months time will not be determined by what you do for the next seven hours, or the next seven days, but by how much exercise you do over the course of the next seven months. So missing a few exercise sessions here and there is okay – what you need to avoid is one missed exercise session snowballing into a complete break. Remember, the key to success is to be consistent – so if you are consistent with your exercise 80% of the time you will lose weight and body fat.

Body Blitz Tip

Stop beating yourself up – if you overindulge one day do not drastically deprive yourself and fast the next. Instead, eat a little less than normal and boost your accumulated activity and structured exercise.

BODY BLITZ CONSISTENCY MAKEOVER

Anna works hard and plays hard. She is a busy 28-year-old executive who has a hectic social life and a demanding job. Before she embarked on the Body Blitz Plan she was experiencing a lot of frustration with her weight despite going to the gym and following a 'diet'. So let's have a look at Anna's pre-Body Blitz eating habits – here are three typical days in Anna's life:

Sunday

breakfast	cup of herbal tea
lunch	mushrooms fried in olive oil; 3 slices of soda bread; green salad with lettuce, tomatoes, peppers and rocket
mid-afternoon snack	large packet of crisps
dinner	low-fat tomato and basil soup; 3 slices of soda bread

Monday

breakfast	cup of herbal tea
lunch	large jacket potato with cottage cheese; small green salad with tomatoes and grated carrots
mid-afternoon snack	cup of herbal tea
dinner	bowl of low-fat tomato and basil soup; smoked mackerel salad; 3 slices of soda bread

Tuesday

breakfast	fruit salad with pineapple, melon, apple and grapes; sesame seed bagel
mid-morning	cappuccino and a croissant
lunch	pasta, pesto and parmesan salad; low-fat chocolate and ginger muffin
mid-afternoon snack	2 chocolate biscuits; handful of little cheesy biscuits
dinner	Thai restaurant – meal shared between two: chicken satay, fish cakes, prawns, mussels, chicken drumstick, Pad Thai, boiled rice, green chicken curry, sizzling seafood platter
	after-dinner mint; half bottle of red wine

Anna was a classic erratic. Her calorie and nutrient intake swung between extremes, leaving her devoid of energy and unable to reach her weight loss targets. A look at Anna's diet diary shows she ate roughly 1,200 calories on Monday compared to a WHOPPING 3,500 calories on Tuesday! It's no surprise that by Wednesday morning Anna didn't feel like she had achieved much towards her diet goal! Anna's inconsistent eating meant she was nowhere near the 80–20 rule's 500 calorie cushion. Here is what Anna says:

'I felt such horror when I first started to record what I was eating. All the peaks and troughs in those figures were enough to put me off fat for life! When I started to put the **80-20 rule** into practice and balance out my calorie and fat intake, I really began to feel the difference.'

ANNA'S MAKEOVER MENU

Anna's makeover involved putting together a plan that fitted with her busy life. She needed to be more organized about her meals and a little thought soon paid huge dividends. Breakfast started to become a regular part of her daily meal plan and the **starch curfew** was a great success to help stabilize her overall calorie intake.

breakfast (8.15 a.m. before leaving for work)	fruit smoothie – made from 250ml soya milk, a selection of fruit including a banana and one tablespoon of wheatgerm; a plain bagel
mid-morning	piece of fruit
lunch (from work canteen)	rice and vegetable stir-fry, or chicken and salad stuffed tortilla, or pasta with a tomato based sauce (large portion – Anna's own words!)
mid-afternoon snack	yoghurt, or piece of fruit, or a shop-bought fruit smoothie
dinner	salmon steaks with yoghurt and dill dressing with a green salad and tomatoes (no dressing)
post-dinner	6 almonds or piece of fruit

ANNA'S VERDICT

So what did Anna really think about her Body Blitz makeover:

The Body Blitz smoothies are great for breakfast – I really look forward to them and feel great because I know they give me a healthy start to my day. Introducing a starch curfew was obviously a huge change in my diet, but boy does it work! In general I now take a lot more care over my evening meal and I find I am eating a much more varied diet. And it really works well for me at home and with all my eating out at restaurants. I am enjoying cooking for myself and find it doesn't really take too much more effort to grill a piece of chicken or salmon than it does to boil a pan of water for pasta.

To begin with I did find it a bit tough reducing my overall fat intake – especially giving up my chocolate biscuits and cheese – but the results speak for themselves. These days when I do eat 'naughty food' I no longer feel too guilty and I certainly don't feel like a failure. I know that my diet is sensible and the fact that I have dropped nearly three dress sizes speaks for itself. I feel fantastic!

So how did Anna do?

Over four months Anna dropped three dress sizes, she lost three inches off her belly button and waist measurements, three inches off her hip and thigh measurements and a total of fifteen pounds of body fat. Anna feels fitter and healthier than she has done for a long time and she certainly still lives her life to the full.

Never Eat on Two Feet!

How many times do you slip something into your mouth without even realizing it? Maybe you are in the kitchen and you are popping food into your mouth while you cook or you are walking past a plate of biscuits or sweets and grabbing a couple as you go – and before you know it you have munched your way through 500 calories! And this is without even sitting down and really appreciating your food. So to help you avoid snacking make sure you always sit down to eat. Remember the mantra: Never eat on two feet! You'll be surprised what a difference it can make.

DOES YOUR LIFESTYLE TRIP YOU UP?

We have now learnt how to apply the **80–20 rule** and seen how we can have a more relaxed approach to diet and fitness just so long as we are consistent. But in real life there will always be times when we cannot help going overboard – those big nights out, birthday celebrations, Christmas festivities and holidays, for starters. And on a day to day level there are also situations that lead us into temptation.

Everyone has different triggers that prompt them to overeat or eat all the wrong foods. Below are some common trigger activities, cues and locations – I am sure at least two or three of these are familiar to you. **Identifying your triggers** is a key step to achieving consistency and learning how to apply **damage limitation** to your Body Blitz Plan.

IDENTIFYING YOUR TRIGGERS

boredom	watching TV	need a reward	tired
cold	in the kitchen	preparing food	clearing food away
social events	birthdays	feeling low and need to be cheered up	feeding the children
time of day	menstrual cycle	binge eating after a night on the town	it's the weekend!
feeling frustrated at work	eating out at restaurants	'I've been good all day so I'll treat myself'	thinking you can overeat after exercise
finishing chores so you feel you deserve a cup of tea and something to eat	picking the children up from school	having a box of chocolates in the house knowing they are there waiting to be eaten	being on holiday
lonely	long car journey	losing your will power when drinking with friends	food shopping when you are hungry
friends who tempt you with goodies	mid-afternoon sugar cravings	biscuits at work	comfort eating

So as you can see from the box above, there are lots of different situations that can act as triggers. We all have a different trigger profile – the challenge for you is to be honest with yourself and really get to know your own profile. Then you will be able to take charge of your triggers rather than your triggers taking charge of you.

You need to understand what prompts you to eat unwisely, whether this is overeating or selecting less healthy choices. Often your perception of a situation, a sequence of events or simply the time of day can act as a cue for you to either eat when you don't need to or to eat inappropriate foods. This I term 'head hunger'. By developing an understanding of the events that act as a trigger for you to eat inappropriately you can identify between 'head hunger' and 'genuine hunger'. You can then start to take control of your actions and develop eating patterns that not only help you reduce excess fat intake and calories BUT also keep your energy levels well fuelled.

DAMAGE LIMITATION STRATEGIES

If from time to time you know that your lifestyle isn't going to fit into your Body Blitz Plan, don't despair. The plan has built in strategies, which allow you to balance things out over time. **Damage limitation** means being realistic about your own habits. It applies to both your fitness and your diet.

TOO BUSY TO GO TO THE GYM

There will always be times when you just can't get to the gym – maybe you're too tired or maybe you don't have the spare time. Instead of despairing that all is lost, the Body Blitz Plan provides ways for you to burn calories any time, any place, anywhere! As we discussed in Step Four, even if you aren't able to take part in a **structured exercise** class or gym session, long-term you can more than make up for the calories you would have burned by **accumulating physical activity** as part of your normal working day.

Just by taking the stairs instead of the elevator, by going on foot to post that letter or simply by putting a bit of extra oomph into your regular walking pace, you can tot up a surprising amount of extra calories burned by the end of the week.

Every Little Bit Helps!

Natasha was suffering from weight gain in her middle years. She had always struggled with her weight but had now resigned herself to the fact that nothing would ever work. Here is her story:

> *I started the Body Blitz Plan when I was menopausal with the disadvantages of weight gain and being very unfit. The understanding of accumulated activity has really helped. If I couldn't get to a class or gym I stopped beating myself up over it and instead took an alternative like a brisk walk, cycling to the shops or doing my housework with extra vigour. And when I do go to the gym, I religiously park my car furthest away from the entrance as I know even that extra little walk will count. It seems to have become a way of life without too much effort. I now have more energy, a spring in my step, awareness of my lifestyle and everybody thinks I look so well.*

So how did she do?

Natasha has lost a stone and a total loss of eight inches around her body.

WHEN IT IS DIFFICULT TO SAY 'NO'!

If you are following the Body Blitz Plan you will be trying to keep to a **starch curfew**. But some nights starch-free is just not possible. Perhaps you are going to eat at a friend's house and you know pasta is her favourite, or you are going to an Indian restaurant (lucky you!) where unless you stick to salads, you most definitely will want some starchy rice or bread to mop up your lamb pasanda. Here are some damage limitation suggestions to help you cope with a wide range of situations:

OPTION 1: PORTION CONTROL

If you are faced with a meal that is high in starches and fats, you can use **portion control** to make sure that all is not lost. **Portion control** allows you enjoy high calorie foods without having to worry too much about consuming excessive calories and fat grams. By making sure your portion size is limited, you can be assured that you have limited your calorie and fat gram intake without having had to say 'no', getting embarrassed or offending your hosts.

Portion control can be achieved by using a smaller plate than usual, by serving a smaller portion than you usually would take, or simply by not quite finishing the portion on your plate.

OPTION 2: STARCH-FREE ZONE

On days when the **starch curfew** is out of the question – perhaps you know in advance that you will be eating starch at dinner – you can limit the damage done to your Body Blitz Plan by bringing in the **starch-free zone**.

The **starch-free zone** shouldn't be necessary too often but you will find it a useful support tool to your healthy eating plans. As I explained in Step One, the **starch-free zone** means no bread, pasta, rice, potatoes or cereal in your midday meal. This then gives you the freedom to consume starch in your evening meal. It has all the benefits of the basic starch curfew but gives you the flexibility to accommodate an evening meal situation where you may not be able to go starch-free. Situations such as eating at friends' houses, a special buffet party, pancake day or maybe those times when you are eating out for both lunch and dinner, are all ideal times to apply the **starch-free zone**. Here are some examples of how to put the **starch-free zone** into practice:

Scenario	Body Blitz Advice
eating at a friend's home	Go starch-free at lunchtime.
a special buffet party	Select starch-free options wherever possible. Have a fruit smoothie before going to party to curb appetite.
eating in a restaurant for lunch and dinner	Consider which venue it is easier to go starch-free – generally it is easier to do it at lunchtime as it limits any difficulties you may experience later.
	Have fruit for breakfast to help save some calories.

Tips from Successful Body Blitzers

Paula:

Always keep in the car sesame ryvita with half-fat cream cheese and of course a bottle of water. This will help you avoid snacking on crisps and chocolate during long journeys.

Lucy:

When I go to restaurants I find I overeat, especially when I look at the men sitting with me. Being only 5 foot 2 they are always much bigger than me. I always used to eat as much as them – now I watch what they eat and I aim to eat about 25% less food on my plate than they do.

Julie:

If you are prone to over-indulging on family comfort foods don't just put them away, cling wrap, seal, bolt or hide them! Do whatever you have to do to put a time and distance parameter between you and temptation. For example, a very effective strategy for me is to put the food in the basement where the ironing is!

BODY BLITZ SUCCESS STORY

Jill had been a heavy smoker for over 40 years – not just social smoking but 30–40 cigarettes a day. A couple of years ago she successfully gave up smoking which she was delighted about but within a year she had gained two stone in weight. Here is her story:

I knew that I would probably gain weight if I stopped smoking and this had always been my excuse for not quitting. But my son and I always pledged that if he gave up smoking so would I, so when he successfully kicked the habit a couple of years ago I decided to give up as well – and after some effort, I was successful too. Wonderful – I was free of this terrible habit. But as I had feared, I ended up eating more to compensate for not smoking. I ate everything bad and lovely, not sweet things but gorgeous savouries – sausage rolls, quiche lorraine, pizzas and freshly baked bread and butter.

Something had to be done so I embarked on the Body Blitz Plan and well, after 10 weeks my life, looks and body have changed. I am now very aware of eating well and drinking loads of water every day – and the gym has become my second home. I strut quickly through space from A to B, always holding my back straight. My deportment is like it used to be when I was a young, as is my skin. As I have always been a businesswoman, I have in the past poo-pooed the idea of exercise and I have never taken any notice of eating properly – always putting stress and tiredness down to age. I now make time every other day at the gym for the new Jill.

The Body Blitz's starch curfew is so sensible and I try to keep to the 5 p.m cut off – of course it is not always possible, but I feel confident with the other strategies I have learnt to make everything work for me and my lifestyle. Again, with this guilt thing all us ladies have, it is very comforting to learn from the Body Blitz Plan that weight loss works over one week. I know this sounds silly, but I have always thought that if

I had a bad day – eating 'bad' foods – I might as well give up altogether. The Body Blitz Plan has made me realize that I have not blown it and by being careful during the week, that one day was not the end of the world and it could be compensated for.

I have lost inches, but most important to me, I have reshaped my body and lost the inches from my 'problem' areas – my thighs and stomach. I have put some effort into this but I am most definitely not a Miss Goody Two Shoes! I really do feel happy and in control of my energy levels and my body fat – and people say I have never looked better!

A FINAL WORD

Being consistent does not mean you have to wear your diet hat all the time. In fact, with the Body Blitz Plan you should feel in control to enjoy your food *and* achieve your weight and body fat goals. Remember, if you can stick to the Body Blitz Plan for 80% of the time you have succeeded! Knowing how to make **damage limitation** work for you will allow you to still live your life to the full and have fun with all the different situations that can get in the way of your good intentions. Keep going – you *can* make this work for you!

Body Blitz Active Action Points:

- Make sure you keep to your starch curfew and remember the other nutritional strategies discussed earlier – and be consistent! Remember the 80–20 rule!
- Identify the triggers that prompt you to eat unwisely so you can make healthier food choices in the future.
- Plan ahead to identify those times when it may be hard to be consistent. If you are aware of these situations you can prepare yourself with the **Body Blitz damage limitation** strategies.

PART III: BODY BLITZ GOOD FOOD GUIDE

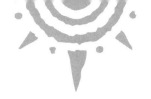

CHAPTER EIGHT

Eating Out

Eating out in a restaurant is about relaxing and enjoying your food and company – you don't want to spend your evening worrying about what is on the menu because you are on a diet. This is where the **starch curfew** is different to a lot of other diets – it gives you the freedom to enjoy your meal, guilt free! By saying no to starches in your evening meal, you can relax and enjoy a wide range of other foods on the menu. Following are some suggestions of good dishes to choose when you are eating in a variety of restaurants – all the dishes listed are healthy and starch-free alternatives. You will probably be surprised to see just how much choice you have. I have also included some general tips for your midday meal.

I have not listed any suggestions for desserts – when you eat a dessert you pile on the extra calories without really needing them. Try waiting 20 minutes before saying yes to a sweet course to establish whether you are still truly hungry. If you decide you do want one, select fresh fruit and sorbets – they are the healthiest choices. Alternatively, opt for a peppermint tea to aid your digestion.

Remember, if you really know you are not going to be able to operate the **starch curfew**, you can always use the **starch-free zone** at lunchtime.

ITALIAN

Although we tend to think that pasta and pizza dishes dominate an Italian menu, you can often find grilled chicken and fish on the menu – both are good choices either at lunchtime or in your evening meal.

If you are eating in an Italian restaurant at lunchtime, order a starter portion of pasta with a tomato-based rather than cream sauce or a small thin crust pizza. Avoid cheese and salami meat toppings on pizzas and say no to the garlic bread.

If you are eating Italian food in the evening, here are some good starch-free dishes to choose from the menu.

Starters:

parma ham with figs or melon

tomato and mozzarella salad (request without olive oil)

tuna and bean salad

gazpacho soup – although originally a Spanish dish you will often find this favourite on Italian menus

Main Courses:

any grilled meat or poultry, for example, pollo cacciatore (chicken with tomato sauce) or vitello scallopine napoletana (veal with tomato sauce)

any fish dish, for example, mixed fish salad or calamari

INDIAN

Spicy Indian meals can be a great choice because even a small portion can satisfy your taste buds! However, be careful because many dishes are full of fat. Go easy on the vegetable side dishes as they can be laden with ghee (clarified butter high in saturated fat), and select chicken or prawn dishes rather than beef or lamb dishes to save some calories.

If you are eating your midday meal in an Indian restaurant, remember that the starchy naan bread and rice accompaniments can boost unwanted calories. Select plain boiled rice rather than pilau rice and choose chappati as opposed to naan bread.

Here are some delicious starch-free dishes to choose for your evening meal.

Starters:

cucumber raita

chicken sashlik

tomato sambal

onion sambal

mulligatawny soup

Main Courses:

chicken tikka

tandoori chicken

tandoori king prawns

tandoori mixed grill

bhuna dishes baked with tomato and onions

chicken jalfrezi

vegetable curry

THAI

There are generally plenty of healthy choices on a Thai menu and the portions tend to be reasonably small. Thai salad dressings are great – often made with lime or lemon juice mixed with fish sauce and a little sugar. If eating chicken satay, go easy on the peanut sauce because it is laden with calories. Also, avoid coconut milk and all cream dishes.

If you are eating Thai food at lunchtime there are many delicious Thai spiced soups to enjoy which are made with stock and prawns or chicken with rice noodles and vegetables. These are filling and satisfying soups – and the addition of the starchy noodles fuels you with energy for the afternoon.

If you are eating in a Thai restaurant in the evening, here are some good starch-free dishes to choose:

Starters:

tom yam gung (hot and sour soup with prawns)

gai tom ke (chicken, coconut and galangel soup)

Main Courses:

Thai beef salad

yam talay (tasty seafood salad)

pla manow (fish with lemon sauce)

normai pad kai (pork with bamboo shoots)

moo pad king (pork with ginger)

ENGLISH

Ask anyone to name a couple of typical English dishes and steak and kidney pies and spongy puddings will probably pop into their mind! Not great dishes if you are trying to say no to starches! With a little care however it is possible to navigate your way around the menu and eat very healthily and happily.

For lunch, choose an open sandwich instead of the traditional closed sandwiches – a great combination is a slice of wholemeal bread spread with a little cranberry sauce, topped with a pile of salad greens, grated carrot and a grilled chicken breast or chicken or turkey slices. If grabbing something from a café opt for a ham roll (and eat only one piece of the roll) rather than a cheese and tomato sandwich. A poached egg on toast with a couple of grilled tomatoes is another great way to get a good balance of starch and protein at lunchtime.

Here are some delicious suggestions for your evening meal:

Starters:

soup – but steer clear of creamy varieties. Say no to the bread roll that accompanies it

smoked salmon – say no to the bread and eat with salad garnish

prawn cocktail with a little dressing

Main Courses:

select roast chicken and turkey rather than cuts of beef, lamb and pork. Remember not to eat the skin

select casseroles such as venison in red wine, chicken with vegetables and pork and apple. Say no to the potatoes and ask for extra vegetables

grilled gammon steak with pineapple and salad – make sure you cut off the visible fat before you eat it

chargrilled salmon with salad – ask for it not to be served drenched in butter!

AMERICAN

The main challenge of eating out US-style is the size of the portions. This is where **portion control** comes in! So although offers such as 'eat all you like' can be a good deal, in terms of the Body Blitz Plan you are going to have to assert a little self discipline!

Everyone loves burgers (unless you are vegetarian!) and a small hamburger (no cheese, no mayonnaise) with a salad garnish contains just 250 calories, so you don't have to say no to burgers at lunchtime. It is when you start adding all the extras that the story changes. American restaurants do great soup and salad bars at lunchtimes – they also do great dressings and they love to put loads of sauces, dips and dressings on all their dishes! So 'help-yourself' salad bars can be great but watch out for the creamy dressings, bacon pieces, croutons and grated cheese. Instead, enjoy the crunchy vegetables such as carrots, broccoli and celery, pile up your plate with water-dense vegetables such as tomatoes, lettuce and cucumber, and enjoy a little olive oil dressing.

Here are some starch-free suggestions for your evening meal:

Starters:

vegetable crudites with salsa dip • mixed salad

a spicy virgin bloody mary – this will satisfy your taste buds and curb your appetite

corn on the cob (request no butter) • vegetable soup

Main Courses:

all steaks: rump, fillet and sirloin contain less than 325 calories per 240g portion. Eat with salad but chop off the visible fat

burgers (say no to the bun) and eat with extra relish and salad toppings

roast quarter chicken (no skin)

chargrilled jerk chicken salad

Cajun grilled prawns with spinach salad

CHINESE

Traditional Chinese cuisine is low in fat but be careful when eating Chinese food from commercial restaurants and takeaways – a lot of the food is deep fried or cooked in excess oil and this can really add on calories. Also, the monosodium glutamate can make you feel bloated and thirsty after your meal as well as the following day. Remember, you can ask to have your food prepared without the MSG.

I am a big fan of soups for lunch – they are filling, nourishing and can be eaten on the run. Bean curd broth is an excellent health choice and the won ton soup (chicken and dumplings) is great if you want something a little more substantial. If you feel like something other than soup, prawn or chicken chop suey is a good lunchtime choice.

If you are eating Chinese food in the evening, here are some delicious starch-free suggestions:

Starters:

hot and sour soup

crab and sweet corn soup

chicken noodle soup

chicken and sweet corn soup

Main Courses:

chicken and stir-fried vegetables

steamed vegetables

pork and pineapple

steamed bok cho (green cabbage) in oyster sauce

tofu and steamed vegetables

steamed fish with ginger and spring onion

chicken and black bean sauce

king prawns with Chinese vegetables

GREEK

Grilled meat and fish and delicious low calorie vegetables such as tomatoes, aubergines, peppers and olives tend to form the base of Greek food. However, be careful of the amount of olive oil you are consuming as often these dishes arrive swimming in the stuff. While good for the heart remember it still contributes to the calories.

A lunchtime snack of taramasalata and pitta bread may seem appealing but be careful how much you eat – taramasalata is laiden with hidden fat. It is better to choose dolmades (stuffed vine leaves) or select one of the starter suggestions below. My favourite is a small greek salad with grilled sardines and a small pitta bread. Or if you fancy something lighter try the avgolemono (chicken and lemon soup).

Here are some good starch-free suggestions for your evening meal.

Starters:
> *olives*
> *hummus*
> *grilled sardines*
> *avgolemono*
> *tzatziki (natural yoghurt with cucumber and mint)*

Main Courses:
> *marinated calamari – drain off the oil*
> *keftedes (meatballs)*
> *traditional Greek feta cheese salad – but ask for the olive oil dressing on the side*
> *grilled lamb and pepper kebab*
> *fish baked in tomato sauce*
> *kleftiko (very slow roasted lamb on bone)*
> *souvlakia (lamb grilled on skewers)*

FRENCH

When eating out French-style watch out for the butter, oil and cream – and of course the customary basket of baguettes. Remember, you can always ask them not to bring bread to the table if you know you will find it hard to resist!

Instead of opting for a croque monsieur at lunchtime try a lobster bisque or bouillabaisse (fish soup) with a side salad or a starter portion of moules marinieres. Traditional moules marinieres is mussels cooked with dry white wine, onion, garlic, parsley and thyme, but some restaurants add cream so check first and ask for it without. The added bonus of moules is the time it takes to navigate your moules shells will give your stomach time to tell you when it is full!

If you are eating French food in the evening, here are some tasty starch-free dishes to choose from the menu.

Starters:

French onion soup

salade niçoise (leave the potatoes and ask for the dressing on the side)

bouillabaisse – say no to the bread spread with rouille

lobster bisque

Main Courses:

grilled dover sole or trout

steak tartare

moules marinieres

ratatouille

chicken chasseur

salmon in red wine

coq au vin

steak au poivre

JAPANESE

Traditional Japanese cuisine is based on fish, raw vegetables, noodles and rice – with very little meat – and is renowned for being healthy. The fish is often served raw and if you have not tried it, you will probably be surprised how tasty it is.

Japanese cuisine is becoming increasingly popular at lunchtime instead of our traditional sandwich. Sushi boxes can now be found in most supermarkets and sandwich bars and they make a tasty lunch offering a good balance of protein and starch as well as being naturally low in saturated fat and calories. You will find them a great way to satisfy you and fuel you with energy for the afternoon.

For your evening meal you can enjoy teppan dishes which are cooked on a griddle, or why not try raw or steamed tofu or sashimi which is raw fish accompanied by grated white cabbage.

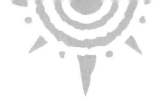

CHAPTER NINE

Eating In

This chapter is full of ideas for your Body Blitz meals when eating at home, showing you how easy it can be to incorporate the Body Blitz diet into your life. Maybe you just want to cook a quick meal for yourself, or you have a hungry family to feed, or you have invited some friends over for dinner – whatever the occasion, you will find a recipe to suit it! Following is a collection of meat, fish and vegetarian recipes for lunchtime and your evening meal. All the recipes are low in fat and calories and provide you with the right balance of nutrients at the right time of the day. The emphasis of Body Blitz cooking is on healthy dishes that are easy to cook as well as appetizing and enjoyable to eat.

BE PREPARED

Before you begin Body Blitz cooking it is important to be prepared. You need to make sure you have a sufficiently stocked storecupboard so you have the right ingredients on hand when you need them.

Your Body Blitz storecupboard should always contain a variety of grains and starch sources such as bread, cereal, rice and pasta – this will provide you with a good range of nutrients and dietary fibres. Porridge oats should be a staple item in your storecupboard – when you eat porridge at breakfast it provides you with a great source of slow energy releasing carbohydrates which set you up for the day. Wheatgerm is another highly nutritious ingredient that is a must-have in your Body Blitz kitchen – it can be added to smoothies or used to top cereals as well as being an ingredient in its own right.

FRUIT AND VEGETABLES

Don't worry if you don't always manage to buy fresh fruit and vegetables – just make sure you have tins of fruit (in natural fruit juice) and vegetables (preferably in water with no added sugar or salt) on hand. It is best to buy water-dense fruit and vegetables such as spinach, cucumbers, tomatoes, peppers, strawberries and melons as they are low in calories and they can help to hydrate you. Frozen fruit and vegetables are very useful to store in the freezer – as we have already seen, frozen fruit makes a great addition to our smoothies. Next time you are in your local supermarket, check out the frozen fruit and veg aisle. And remember, you can always freeze your overripe bananas – peel and cut into chunks, place in small freezer bags and pop in the freezer for use at a later date.

DRIED FRUIT

Dried fruit is naturally low in fat, a good source of dietary fibre and iron, and it can give you a good natural sugar energy boost – but beware of the calories. A 50g bag of pineapple, papaya or mango provides 270 calories and a 50g bag of apricots provides 165 calories – so buy little individual bags to avoid a big bag of dried apricots suddenly disappearing in one go!

DAIRY PRODUCTS

When buying dairy products, always select the low-fat varieties wherever possible. Fromage frais, for example, is a great low-fat alternative to yoghurt. Also, get into the habit of buying organic soya milk and organic tofu. Both tofu and soya milk are low in calories and highly nutritious; they are also good sources of phyto-oestrogens, which have been shown to have a protective effect against some reproductive cancers.

MEAT, FISH AND POULTRY

When buying your fresh meat, fish and poultry buy in bulk and then freeze in smaller portions for convenience – this works particularly well with chicken breasts and fish fillets. And don't forget about tinned sources of fish like canned pilchards, sardines, pink salmon and tuna, which can make handy economical protein sources for lunch and supper. They are also an excellent source of omega-3 essential fats: remember the Body Blitz Plan is not about cutting out all fat from your diet – rather it is about consuming the right types of fats. Pre-cut wafer thin sandwich meats are also great to have on hand for snacks. Try lean ham, chicken and turkey for the lowest calorie value and saturated fat content.

PULSES AND BEANS

Pulses such as butter beans, chick peas and kidney beans are a key ingredient in the Body Blitz diet – especially if you are a vegetarian – so stock up on them. They provide an excellent source of dietary fibre as well as being good sources of minerals and B-complex vitamins; they also help control blood sugar levels and lower blood cholesterol levels. You can either buy pulses dried or in tins – dried pulses need soaking for anything up to five hours, so if you are short of time you may prefer to use the tinned variety.

SEEDS AND NUTS

Your storecupboard should also always contain seeds and nuts, which are an excellent source of protein. Nuts can add a great crunch element to your diet and they provide an excellent source of vitamin E as well as other minerals and vitamins including vitamin B. But beware – these healthy additions to your diet have a high calorie content: 100g of cashews, pistachios, almonds or hazelnuts contain over 550 calories and more than 45g of fat. So be careful how many nuts you nibble! Seeds such as linseeds, sesame, sunflower and pumpkin are excellent sources of essential fats. Linseeds, for example, are great added to smoothies, porridge and casseroles – crush them with a pestle and mortar to release their beneficial health properties.

OILS

Monounsaturated oils such as olive oil are a better choice to cook with than polyunsaturated oils as they are more stable when heated at higher temperatures. Cold pressed oils such as flax seed oil (found in the fridge section of health food shops) is a good source of omega-3 oils – however it is not stable when heated so do not use for cooking. Instead, keep it in the fridge and use as a dressing on salads. Don't overlook flavoured vinegars as they can add a variety of tastes to low-fat dressings, marinades and seasonings. If you are able to invest in good quality vinegars your taste buds will really notice the difference.

While the aim of the Body Blitz diet is to limit the use of additional sugar in your cooking, all storecupboards will contain some sugar. You may wish to use an artificial sweetener such as aspartame to keep your calorie content down. But beware – some studies have shown that a high intake of these artificial sweeteners can cause additional carbohydrate cravings and have harmful effects on health. So you may prefer to use the natural thing – but use sparingly! Natural fruit spreads and fresh honeycomb are preferable over commercial high sugar jams.

Finally, don't forget to stock up on fresh herbs. Buy pots of herbs from your supermarket, pop them on your window ledge and let them grow. As you will see from the following recipes, they are a must-have ingredient in the Body Blitz storecupboard.

STARCH CURFEW DINNERS

Here is a selection of starch-free recipes for your evening meal. The emphasis of the dishes is on protein, essential fats, low-fat dairy products and vegetables. All starch curfew dinners also work well as starch-free zone lunches.

At the end of each recipe you will see the calorie and fat content of each dish.

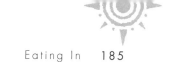

MEAT DISHES

LAMB AND VEGETABLE HOT-POT

Serves 4

200g onions

200g carrots

200g swede or turnip

200g parsnip

1 tablespoon vegetable oil

500g cubed lamb stewing steak

340ml bitter beer (large can)

1 bay leaf or bouquet garni

salt and pepper, to taste

Preheat the oven to 150°C/300°F. Peel all the vegetables and cut them into bite-sized pieces. In a large non-stick frying pan, heat the oil and add the cubed lamb. Cook over a high heat, stirring frequently until the meat is brown on the outside but not cooked through. Transfer to an oven-proof lidded casserole dish.

Add the vegetable pieces to the frying pan, working in batches if necessary, and cook until just beginning to brown. Transfer the vegetables to the casserole and stir well. Pour in the beer, then add the bay leaf or bouquet garni and season generously with salt and pepper. Cover the casserole and place in the oven for 2 hours. Halfway through the cooking time remove the lid and stir. The hot-pot is done when the meat and vegetables are very tender and most of the beer has been absorbed. Remove the bay leaf or bouquet garni and season again to taste before serving.

calories per serving: 188   fat grams per serving: 10

GRILLED STEAKS WITH ASPARAGUS AND BALSAMIC SHALLOTS

Serves 2   2 lean beef steaks

2 cloves garlic

200g shallots

4 tablespoons balsamic vinegar

1 crumpled bay leaf

200g asparagus

1 teaspoon flaked sea salt, plus extra to season

1 teaspoon olive oil

freshly ground black pepper

Preheat the oven to 180°C/350°F. Place the steaks in a non-corrosive dish. Crush the garlic finely and rub it over the steaks. Season generously with sea salt and pepper and set aside to marinate for 30–60 minutes.

Peel the shallots and trim the ends. Halve lengthways and place in a small oven-proof dish in which the shallots fit snugly – this is important. In a small bowl, combine the balsamic vinegar with 100ml of water and pour it over the shallots. Add the bay leaf and place in the hot oven for 30 minutes.

Meanwhile, place the olive oil in another oven-proof dish and add the trimmed asparagus. Rub the asparagus with the oil then sprinkle with the sea salt and black pepper. When the shallots have been cooking for 30 minutes, remove them from the oven and stir thoroughly. Return the shallots to the oven, placing the dish of asparagus in the oven at the same time and cook for another 20 minutes.

Ten minutes before the end of cooking the asparagus and shallots, heat a griddle over a very high heat until smoking. Use kitchen paper to wipe the crushed garlic from the steaks, then add them to the pan. Immediately turn the heat down to medium-low and cook for 1–2 minutes on each side, depending on how thoroughly you like steak cooked.

Remove the shallots and asparagus from the oven and arrange on serving plates. Top with the steak and serve accompanied by a chutney or mustard, if desired.

calories per serving: 379   fat grams per serving: 16

THAI BEEF SALAD

Serves 2   *For the beef:*
2 lean beef steaks
juice of 1 lime
1 tablespoon soy sauce

For the salad:
150g tomatoes
100g celery
100g spring onions
100g carrot
15g coriander

For the dressing:
1–2 small red chillies • 1 clove garlic
1 teaspoon fish sauce
1/2 teaspoon palm sugar, brown sugar or honey

Place the steaks in a non-corrosive dish. Set aside 2 tablespoons of the lime juice in a small bowl and pour the remainder over the steaks. Add the soy sauce to the meat and set aside to marinate for 30–60 minutes.

Meanwhile, to make the salad, put a kettle of water on to boil. Using a small knife, score a cross in the base of each tomato. Place them in a heat-proof bowl and cover with the boiled water. Leave to stand for 1–2 minutes, then drain and refresh under cold water. When cool, peel and core the tomatoes. Discard the seeds and cut the flesh into strips. De-string the celery and cut into matchsticks. Cut the spring onions into fine strips. Use a vegetable peeler to cut the carrot into ribbons. Combine the vegetables in a salad bowl. Roughly chop the coriander, including the tender stalks, and stir it into the vegetables.

To make the salad dressing, crush the chillies and garlic together using a pestle and mortar to make a paste. Stir in the reserved 2 tablespoon of lime juice, plus the fish sauce and sugar or honey.

Heat a griddle over a very high heat for about 5 minutes or until very hot and smoking. Add the marinated steaks and immediately turn the heat down to medium-low. Cook for 1–2 minutes on each side, depending on how thoroughly you like steak cooked.

Pour the salad dressing over the vegetables and toss well. Divide amongst serving plates and top with the cooked steak – you can cut the steak into strips first if you prefer.

calories per serving: 444   fat grams per serving: 19

SPICY SAUSAGE WITH CHERRY TOMATO SAUCE AND BROCCOLI CHILLI PESTO

Sausages are generally a high fat food but here is a recipe that uses storecupboard ingredients and the family-favourite sausage to achieve a starch-curfew dinner. Serve with a salad and you have a well-balanced and tasty evening meal.

Serves 2   250g spicy Italian fresh sausages

For the cherry tomato sauce:
1 teaspoon olive oil
300g cherry tomatoes
paprika or cayenne pepper, to taste

For the broccoli chilli pesto:
stem of 1 piece broccoli
3–4 basil leaves • 1–2 green olives
$1/2$ teaspoon dried chilli flakes
salt and pepper, to taste

To make the broccoli chilli pesto, chop the broccoli stem into small pieces. Place in a small saucepan, cover with water and bring to the boil. Simmer for 5–8 minutes or until the broccoli stem is very tender. Drain well, reserving the cooking water, and allow to cool briefly.

Transfer the broccoli to a food processor or blender and add the basil, olives, chilli flakes and a little salt and pepper. Process until smooth, adding just enough of the reserved cooking water to make a spoonable paste. Adjust the seasonings to taste and set aside.

To make the cherry tomato sauce, place the olive oil in a large heavy-based saucepan. Rinse the cherry tomatoes and add them to the pan without letting them dry. Cover the pan and set over a low heat. Cook for about 3 minutes, shaking the pan frequently. Remove the lid and mash the cherry tomatoes a little with a wooden spoon – the mixture should form a sauce but retain some texture. Add the paprika or cayenne, cover the pan again and continue cooking gently for another 5–10 minutes, stirring occasionally.

Meanwhile, preheat the grill to the highest setting. Cook the spicy sausages on a rack set over the grill-pan so that the excess fat drains away during cooking. Turn frequently during cooking – the exact time needed will depend on the thickness of the sausages.

Adjust the seasonings of the cherry tomato sauce to taste then arrange a pool of sauce on the serving plates. Top with the cooked sausages, then add a dollop of the broccoli chilli pesto.

calories per serving: 390   fat grams per serving: 22

CHICKEN DISHES

CHICKEN AND APRICOT TAGINE

Serves 4   8 skinless, boneless chicken thighs

150g dried apricots, chopped

225g onions, chopped

225g mushrooms, chopped

725ml chicken or vegetable stock

a pinch of saffron

a pinch of ginger

a pinch of cumin

salt and pepper, to taste

fresh coriander to garnish (optional)

Place all the ingredients in a large, heavy-based saucepan or casserole dish and bring to the boil. Cover, lower the heat right down and simmer for 45 minutes, stirring occasionally.

When cooked, remove the lid and simmer uncovered until most of the liquid evaporates and you have a thick stew. Adjust the seasoning to taste and serve garnished with fresh coriander if desired.

calories per serving: 259   fat grams per serving: 5

CHILLED CHICKEN SALAD WITH SMOKED PAPRIKA

Serves 2   *For the chicken:*

2 skinless, boneless chicken breasts

vegetable stock or water to cover

a splash of vinegar, white wine or lemon juice

1 bay leaf or bouquet garni

For the salad:

2 red bell peppers • 75g cucumber, sliced or chopped

140g mixed salad leaves

2–3 tablespoons fresh parsley leaves

For the sauce:

125g plain low-fat yoghurt • 2 teaspoons sun-dried tomato paste

1 1/2–2 tablespoons finely chopped fresh herbs such as basil,
    chives, parsley

1 small clove garlic, crushed • 1 tablespoon lemon juice

1/8–1/4 teaspoon smoked paprika, or to taste

salt and pepper, to taste

Place the chicken breasts in a frying pan with the vinegar, white wine or lemon juice and the bay leaf or bouquet garni. Cover with vegetable stock or water and bring to the boil. Lower the heat to a very gentle simmer and cook for 25 minutes until the chicken is done.

Meanwhile, start preparing the salad. Heat the grill to the highest setting and grill the whole red bell peppers until they are blistered and blackened all over. Remove from the heat, place in a bowl and cover with cling-film. Leave to stand for 10 minutes to make the skins easier to remove.

When the chicken is cooked, remove it from the pan and set aside to cool on paper towels. Peel the black skin from the peppers, discard the core and seeds and cut the flesh into strips. Combine in a salad bowl with the cucumber, salad leaves and parsley.

In a small mixing bowl, combine all the ingredients for the sauce. Cube the cooled chicken and stir it into the sauce. Arrange the salad on serving plates, top with the dressed chicken and serve.

calories per serving: 251   fat grams per serving: 6

LIGHT CHICKEN CURRY WITH SPINACH

Serves 2   2 medium-large onions, finely chopped

500ml chicken or vegetable stock

1 large Bramley or other cooking apple, peeled, cored and diced

1 tablespoon sultanas

1 heaped tablespoon garam masala

2 part-boned chicken breasts

140g baby spinach leaves

fresh coriander to garnish; salt and pepper, to taste

a little freshly grated nutmeg (optional)

Place the onions and half the stock in a casserole dish or heavy-based saucepan and bring to a hard boil. Lower the heat, cover and leave to simmer for 15 minutes until the onions are tender. Remove the lid and raise the heat a little. Simmer until the liquid has almost evaporated, then add the apples and sultanas and cook for 5 minutes, stirring occasionally. Add the garam masala and stir to give a thick sauce, then add the chicken and stir until thoroughly coated with the sauce. Pour in the remaining stock and bring to the boil. Cover and lower the heat right down so that the stew simmers very gently for 30 minutes.

Uncover the stew and remove the cooked chicken to a plate. Raise the heat under the pan and simmer until the sauce mixture has reduced to a thick coating consistency. Return the chicken to the pan and add salt and pepper to taste. Allow to heat through briefly.

Meanwhile, place the washed spinach in a large saucepan over a low heat. Cover and cook for 5 minutes, stirring occasionally, until the leaves have wilted. Add salt and pepper to taste, plus some grated nutmeg if desired.

Divide the spinach amongst serving plates. Top with the chicken and sauce and garnish with the fresh coriander.

calories per serving: 402   fat grams per serving: 9

PROVENÇALE-STYLE POACHED CHICKEN WITH VEGETABLES

Serves 2   2 skinless, boneless chicken breasts

725ml chicken stock

4 tablespoons white wine

1 teaspoon herbes de Provence mixture

100g tomatoes

100g broccoli florets

100g courgettes

75g leeks

75g baby carrots

1 tablespoon finely chopped fresh parsley, to garnish

salt and pepper, to taste

Place the chicken breasts in a frying pan with the stock, wine and herbes de Provence. Bring to the boil then cover and simmer gently for 20 minutes.

Meanwhile, put a kettle of water on to boil. Using a small knife, cut a small cross in the base of the tomatoes. Place in a heat-proof bowl and cover with boiling water. Leave to stand for 1–2 minutes, then drain and peel the tomatoes. Discard the seeds, reserving as much of the tomato juice as possible. Cut the flesh into strips and set aside with the juices.

Cut the broccoli, courgettes and leeks into bite-sized pieces. When the chicken has been cooking for 20 minutes, add all the vegetables including the tomato strips and carrots, then season to taste with salt and pepper. Cover and cook for another 5 minutes or until the chicken is fully cooked and the vegetables are just tender.

Transfer the vegetables and chicken to large soup bowls and top with a generous quantity of the broth. Sprinkle with the parsley and serve with knives, forks and soup spoons so that diners can enjoy the broth.

calories per serving: 174   fat grams per serving: 4

FISH DISHES

GRILLED TUNA WITH BEETROOT HUMMUS

Serves 2   *For the fish:*

2 small tuna steaks

1 tablespoon Thai sweet chilli sauce

1 teaspoon sesame oil

For the beetroot hummus:

250g cooked beetroot

400g canned chickpeas

1 teaspoon cumin

1–2 cloves garlic

juice of 1 lemon

1 teaspoon sesame oil

salt and pepper, to taste

For the salad:

100g watercress or rocket leaves

50g salad onions or scallions, finely sliced

Place the tuna in a non-corrosive dish and rub with the chilli sauce and sesame oil. Leave to stand in a cool place for 1–2 hours to marinate.

Meanwhile, place all the ingredients for the hummus in a blender and process to a slightly textured paste. Add just enough water to give the mixture the consistency of thick yoghurt.

When ready to cook the fish, heat a griddle or heavy non-stick frying pan over a high heat until almost smoking. Add the fish and immediately lower the heat to medium-low. Cook the fish for 2 minutes on each side or until done to your liking. Alternatively, cook under an overhead grill heated to high.

Spoon the beetroot hummus onto serving plates and arrange the watercress or rocket and the salad onions next to it. Top the hummus with the tuna and serve.

calories per serving: 467   fat grams per serving: 13

LIME MARINATED GRILLED SALMON WITH SALSA

Serves 2   *For the fish:*

2 small fillets salmon or other oily fish

grated zest and juice of 1 lime

2 teaspoons brown sugar

2 teaspoons olive oil

salt and pepper, to taste

For the salsa:

250g red bell pepper

250g tomatoes

50g mild onion

1 fresh green chilli

1 clove garlic, crushed

1–2 tablespoons fresh lime juice

1–2 tablespoons chopped fresh coriander leaves

Place the salmon in a non-corrosive dish. In a small bowl, combine the lime zest and juice, sugar, olive oil and salt and pepper to taste. Pour over the fish and leave to marinate for at least 30 minutes in a cool place.

Meanwhile, heat the grill to the highest setting. Place the bell peppers and tomatoes under the grill and cook until blistered and blackened all over, turning frequently. Remove each vegetable from the heat as it is done and transfer to a bowl and cover with cling film. Leave to stand for 10 minutes to make the skins easier to remove.

Peel, seed and core the peppers and tomatoes, reserving as many of the tasty juices as possible. Chop the flesh finely and place in a clean bowl with the juices. Finely chop the onion and green chilli and stir them into the salsa, along with the garlic, lime juice and coriander. Season to taste with salt and pepper.

When ready to cook the fish, heat the grill to high and remove the fish from the marinade, discarding the excess marinade. Cook the fish for 2–3 minutes on each side or until done to your liking. Remove from the heat and serve with the salsa.

calories per serving: 425   fat grams per serving: 22

PRAWN, SCALLOP AND PARMA HAM KEBABS WITH PARSLEY SALAD

Serves 4   *For the kebabs:*

8 raw king prawns

8 fresh king scallops

2 cloves garlic, crushed

2 tablespoons chopped fresh basil

juice of 1/2 lemon

1 tablespoon olive oil

12 slices Parma ham or prosciutto crudo

For the salad:

150g fresh parsley

30g pitted black olives

4 spring onions • 1/2 red onion

1 tablespoon lime or lemon juice

300g tomatoes, thickly sliced

200g cucumber, thickly sliced

Clean and de-vein the shellfish as necessary, removing the shells. Place in a non-corrosive bowl with the garlic, basil, lemon juice and olive oil. Add some salt and pepper and set aside to marinate for 15–20 minutes.

Meanwhile, to make the salad, chop the parsley roughly, discarding any coarse stems but retaining the tender ones. Place in a salad bowl. Very finely chop the olives, spring onions and red onion and stir them into the parsley, adding the lime or lemon juice and salt and pepper to taste.

Heat the grill to the highest setting. Gather a slice of ham into a ruffle and thread it onto a metal skewer. Then thread on a scallop and a prawn. Repeat and finish the kebab with another ruffle or ham. Prepare another three metal skewers the same way.

Place the kebabs under the grill and cook for about 5 minutes, turning and basting with the excess marinade frequently. They are ready when the ham is crisp and the shellfish is just cooked.

Meanwhile, lay the slices of tomato and cucumber in a circle on the serving plates. Top each with a mound of parsley salad, then lay a cooked kebab on top. Pour the cooking juices from the grill-pan over the plate as a dressing for the salad.

calories per serving: 206   fat grams per serving: 10

SPICED FISH WITH CAJUN VEGETABLES

Serves 2   *For the spiced fish:*

1 large clove garlic

$1/2$ teaspoon fennel seeds

$1/2$ teaspoon black peppercorns

$1/2$ teaspoon dried mixed herbs

$1/4$ teaspoon cayenne pepper or paprika

a large pinch of salt

1 tablespoon cornmeal

2 skinned halibut fillets

1 tablespoon olive oil

For the Cajun vegetables:

1 green bell pepper, deseeded

1 small onion

1 stick celery

400g canned chopped tomatoes

1 bay leaf

1 teaspoon cayenne pepper or paprika

$1/2$–1 teaspoon molasses or black treacle, or to taste

salt and pepper, to taste

To prepare the Cajun vegetables, finely chop the green bell pepper, onion and celery. Place them in a heavy saucepan with the canned chopped tomatoes, bay leaf, cayenne or paprika, and molasses or black treacle. Add about 4 tablespoons of water and bring the mixture to the boil, stirring. Season to taste with salt and pepper. Cover the pan, then lower the heat right down and simmer gently for 20 minutes.

Begin preparing the spiced fish – use a pestle and mortar to crush the garlic, fennel and peppercorns until fine. Stir in the dried mixed herbs, cayenne or paprika, salt and cornmeal.

When the vegetables have been cooking for 20 minutes, remove the lid and allow to simmer uncovered, stirring constantly, until the mixture is thick and the excess liquid has evaporated. Set aside in a warm place.

Use the spice mixture to coat the fish evenly, pressing it into the flesh. Heat the olive oil in a frying pan over a high heat and cook the coated fish for 90 seconds on each side, or until lightly browned and cooked through.

Divide the vegetable mixture onto the plates and serve the fish on top.

calories per serving: 360   fat grams per serving: 15

VEGETARIAN DINNERS

STEAMED TOFU AND AUBERGINES WITH AROMATIC CHINESE SAUCE

Serves 2
220g plain or smoked tofu

200g aubergine

100g asparagus

100g broccoli

For the sauce:

2 tablespoons soy sauce

2 teaspoons oyster-flavoured sauce

2 teaspoons chilli sauce

2 teaspoons sesame oil

2 spring onions, chopped

Cut the tofu into equal sized blocks. Finely slice the aubergine and cut the asparagus and broccoli into bite-sized pieces. Fill a saucepan with water to a depth of about $2\frac{1}{2}$ cm and place a steamer over the top. Bring the water to the boil. Lay the tofu in the steamer and surround it with the aubergine, broccoli and asparagus. Cover and steam for 5 minutes.

In a small saucepan, combine the soy sauce, oyster sauce, chilli sauce and sesame oil. Bring to the boil and simmer for 2–3 minutes or until the mixture has thickened slightly.

Use a fish slice to transfer the cooked tofu and vegetables to serving plates. Pour the hot sauce over the top and garnish with the chopped spring onions.

calories per serving: 127   fat grams per serving: 11

VEGETABLE AND MISO SOUP WITH TERIYAKI TOFU

Serves 2

For the tofu:
220g tofu
2 tablespoons teriyaki marinade

For the soup:
100g carrot
100g cauliflower
100g broccoli
100g cabbage
400ml vegetable stock
1 tablespoon mirin or sherry
2 tablespoons miso
1 small chilli, sliced
2 spring onions, sliced
1 teaspoon sesame seeds

Cut the tofu into equal sized blocks and rub with the teriyaki marinade. Place in a non-corrosive dish and set aside to marinate for 20 minutes.

Dice the carrot. Cut the cauliflower and broccoli into bite-sized pieces. Shred the cabbage. Place the vegetable stock and mirin or sherry in a large saucepan and bring to the boil. Add the chopped vegetables, stir and simmer for 5 minutes or until the vegetables are cooked.

Remove a ladle of broth from the pot and place in a small bowl. Stir the miso into the bowl of broth, then stir the miso and broth into the soup. Lower the heat under the pan right down – enough to keep the soup warm without letting it boil.

Heat a griddle or non-stick frying pan over a high heat until smoking. Lay the marinated tofu in the pan and immediately turn the heat down to medium-low. Cook for 2 minutes on each side, turning carefully with a fish slice.

Divide the soup amongst serving bowls ensuring each diner has a mixture of vegetables. Top with the cooked tofu, then sprinkle with sliced chilli, chopped spring onions and sesame seeds. Serve hot.

calories per serving: 163   fat grams per serving: 7

MEXICAN BEAN CHILLI

Serves 4   150g black beans

2 dried chipotle chillies

800g canned chopped tomatoes

1 red bell pepper

1 stick celery • 1 small carrot

2 cloves garlic • 1 teaspoon cumin

salt and pepper, to taste

2–3 sprigs fresh coriander

The day before serving, place the black beans in a bowl and cover generously with around 300ml water. Leave to soak overnight.

The next day, drain the black beans. Place in a saucepan and cover with around 300ml of fresh water. Bring to the boil and simmer for 1 hour or until the beans are tender – the exact time will depend on the age of the beans.

Meanwhile, in a small, heavy-based frying pan, toast the dried chillies over a very low heat until fragrant, turning frequently. Transfer to a small bowl. Pour 300ml of boiling water over the toasted chillies and leave to soak for 20 minutes. Remove the chillies from the soaking liquid and remove the cores and seeds. Chop the chillies roughly then return them to the soaking water. Using a hand blender, puree the chillies and soaking water together to give a hot, smoky liquid.

Place the chilli puree in a large saucepan and add the canned tomatoes. Chop the bell pepper, celery and carrot finely and add them to the tomato mixture. Crush the garlic and stir it in with the cumin.

When the beans are tender, drain them and transfer to the tomato mixture. Bring the mixture to a boil, then lower the heat and simmer for 30 minutes or until the chilli is thick and all the flavours have amalgamated. Season to taste with salt and pepper. Serve garnished with the sprigs of fresh coriander.

calories per serving: 100   fat grams per serving: 3

BEAN BURGERS WITH A LIGHT CAESAR-STYLE SALAD

Serves 2

For the bean burgers:
150g cooked or canned black beans or other cooked beans
2 heaped tablespoons finely grated carrot
2 heaped tablespoons finely grated onion
2 tablespoons chopped fresh coriander
salt and pepper, to taste
1 teaspoon olive oil

For the salad dressing:
4 tablespoons low-fat yoghurt
3 tablespoons grated parmesan cheese
6 drops Tabasco sauce
6 drops Worcestershire sauce
1/4 teaspoon mustard
1/2 small clove crushed garlic
1/4 teaspoon black olive paste or 1 anchovy

For the salad:
200g cucumber
250g mixed salad leaves

In a small bowl, mash the beans for the burgers thoroughly. Stir in the carrot, onion and coriander and season to taste with salt and pepper. Shape the mixture into 2 large burgers.

To make the salad dressing, combine the yoghurt, parmesan, Tabasco, Worcestershire sauce, mustard and crushed garlic in a bowl. If using black olive paste, stir it into the dressing; if using anchovy, rinse it thoroughly, pat dry and mince finely before stirring it into the dressing.

To cook the bean burgers, heat the oil in a non-stick frying pan. Place the burgers in the pan and immediately turn the heat down to medium-low. Cook for 2–3 minutes on each side or until crusty and golden brown on the outside. Transfer to a plate lined with paper towel to drain off oil and set aside in a warm place.

Halve the cucumber lengthways and scoop out the seeds using a teaspoon. Cut the flesh into bite-sized pieces and toss in a salad bowl with the mixed salad leaves. Drizzle the dressing over the top. Arrange the dressed salad on serving plates and top with the bean burgers. Serve the bean burgers warm.

calories per serving: 450   fat grams per serving: 23

SPANISH WHITE BEAN STEW

Serves 2   800g cooked or canned white beans such as cannellini or butter beans
1 large green bell pepper
1 large onion
1 large tomato
1 large carrot
1 red or green chilli
vegetable stock, to cover
2 teaspoons olive oil
salt and pepper, to taste

Finely dice all the vegetables. Place in a large saucepan with the drained beans. Stir, then add enough vegetable stock to cover the ingredients. Bring to the boil over a high heat, then lower the heat right down and cover. Simmer for 30 minutes or until the stew is soft, stirring occasionally. Season to taste with salt and pepper. Divide amongst serving bowls and drizzle each bowl with 1 teaspoon olive oil before serving.

calories per serving: 383   fat grams per serving: 8

LENTIL LOAF WITH YELLOW PEPPER SAUCE

Serves 4   *For the loaf:*

125g green lentils

125g yellow split peas

125g chopped onion

1 egg

3 tablespoons olive oil, plus extra for greasing

2 tablespoons chopped fresh parsley

1 tablespoon chopped fresh tarragon

1 large clove garlic

1/2 teaspoon baking powder

1/2 teaspoon salt

For the sauce:

100g tomatoes

4 yellow bell peppers

1 tablespoon chopped basil

2 teaspoons white wine vinegar or sherry vinegar

salt and pepper, to taste

To make the lentil loaf, soak the green lentils and yellow split peas in a generous quantity of water for 4–5 hours or overnight. When ready to cook, preheat the oven to 190°C/375°F and line a loaf tin with kitchen foil, greasing it lightly with olive oil.

Place all the ingredients for the loaf in a food processor and whizz until smooth and combined. Stir by hand halfway through if necessary to help move the ingredients around the bowl of the processor. Pour the lentil mixture into the prepared loaf tin and smooth over the top. Bake in the oven for 45–50 minutes.

Meanwhile, to make the sauce, put a kettle of water on to boil. Use a small sharp knife to cut a cross in the base of the tomatoes and place them in a heat-proof bowl. Cover with the boiling water and leave to stand for 1–2 minutes. Drain and refresh with cold water. When cool, peel and core the tomatoes. Discard the seeds but retain as many juices as possible. Cut the flesh into fine strips and set aside with the juices in a bowl.

Halve, core and deseed the bell peppers. Place them skin-side up on a foil-lined grill-pan and grill for 20 minutes until the skins are black and blistered. Remove the pan from the heat and fold the foil up around the peppers to make a pouch. Leave to stand for 5 minutes so that the skins are easier to remove.

Peel the peppers, discarding the black skins, and transfer the flesh to a blender. Add the vinegar, basil and 1 tablespoon of water and process until smooth. Add more water as necessary to give the consistency of a thick sauce. Transfer the mixture to a small saucepan and add salt and pepper to taste. Heat through gently, then stir in the reserved tomatoes and their juices and keep warm until the lentil loaf is cooked.

Remove the loaf from the oven and cut into slices. Serve with the vegetable sauce poured over the top.

calories per serving: 270   fat grams per serving: 18

ONIONS STUFFED WITH CHARD AND NUTS

Serves 2   4 large onions, about 220g each

100g chard

10g porcini

4 tablespoons low-fat cottage cheese

2 tablespoons chopped walnuts

2 tablespoons parmesan cheese, to sprinkle

salt and pepper, to taste

Peel the onions and trim the bases carefully leaving enough root on the onions to keep the layers together. Place in a large pot and cover generously with water. Cover, bring to the boil and simmer for 45 minutes or until the onions are very tender and sweet. Remove from the liquid and set aside to cool thoroughly.

Use about 100ml of the hot onion cooking water to soak the porcini in a small bowl for 20 minutes. When the onions are cool enough to handle, trim about $2\frac{1}{2}$ cm off the top of each and scoop out most of the innards with a teaspoon, leaving an onion shell 3 layers thick. Finely chop enough of the cooked onion to give 2 tablespoons.

Preheat the oven to 180°C/350°F. Drain the porcini, reserving the soaking liquid, and chop finely. In a frying pan, combine the onion, porcini and 4–6 tablespoons of the mushroom soaking liquid. Cook over a high heat, stirring frequently, until the vegetables begin to soften, then add the chard, season to taste, and continue cooking for 5 minutes or until the leaves have wilted and the mixture is very dry.

Remove the pan from the heat and stir in the cottage cheese and walnuts. Use this mixture to fill the onion shells. Place them in a baking dish small enough to fit them snugly. Sprinkle with parmesan cheese and place in the oven for 10–15 minutes. Serve garnished with black pepper.

calories per serving: 679   fat grams per serving: 47

ASPARAGUS, PEPPER AND COURGETTE OMELETTE

Serves 4

2 onions

1 swede

1 carrot

2 teaspoons olive oil

300g canned asparagus

1 courgette

1 red bell pepper

125g reduced-fat cheddar cheese

4 whole eggs plus 4 egg whites

salt and pepper, to taste

To serve:

200g mixed lettuce leaves

a squeeze of lemon juice

Preheat the oven to 180°C/350°F. Finely slice the onions, swede and carrot. Arrange in a large round ovenproof dish, preferably non-stick, and pour over the oil. Season lightly with salt and pepper. Cover with kitchen foil and bake for 30 minutes until tender.

Drain the asparagus thoroughly. Cut the courgette and bell pepper into sticks a similar size to the asparagus. In a mixing bowl, beat together the whole eggs and egg whites and season lightly with salt and pepper. Gently stir in the cheese.

Remove the dish of vegetables from the oven and remove the foil. Leave the oven on. Arrange the asparagus, courgette and pepper on top of the cooked vegetables like the spokes of a wheel. Pour over the egg mixture and bake uncovered for 15 minutes. Serve at room temperature with green salad leaves dressed with a squeeze of lemon and a little salt and pepper.

calories per serving: 266   fat grams per serving: 17

PUMPKIN AND MUSHROOM STEW

Serves 4   1 large pumpkin, about 30cm diameter

200g onions

200g mushrooms

2 tablespoons olive oil

300ml vegetable stock

6 tablespoons flaked almonds or pine kernels

3 tablespoons low-fat fromage frais

2 tablespoons chopped fresh parsley

salt and pepper, to taste

Peel, core and deseed the pumpkin. Cut the flesh into bite-sized pieces. Slice the onions and mushrooms. Heat the oil in a pot or very large saucepan. Add the onions and stir-fry until golden. Add the pumpkin and continue cooking, stirring frequently, until it begins to brown. Add the mushrooms and cook until they begin to soften.

Pour the vegetable stock into the pan, bring to the boil, then lower the heat and simmer until the pumpkin is tender and the cooking liquid has evaporated.

Meanwhile, in a dry frying pan, toast the almonds or pine kernels over a moderate heat, stirring constantly, until golden brown. Remove to a plate to cool.

When the pumpkin is tender, remove the pan from the heat and stir in the fromage frais and parsley. Generously season to taste with salt and pepper and serve scattered with the toasted nuts.

calories per serving: 348   fat grams per serving: 30

BODY BLITZ LUNCHES

Here is a selection of recipes for your midday meal, which provide a good balance of starch and protein. Some you will find work better to eat at home – others can easily be put in a lunch box to go. By omitting some of the starch accompaniments you can also double these up as starch curfew dinners!

MEXICAN-STYLE WRAPS WITH BEANS, HERBS AND VEGETABLES

Serves 1
100g canned kidney beans

100g canned asparagus

2 tablespoons plain fromage frais

1–2 tablespoons coriander leaves

1 tablespoon flat-leaf parsley

1 tablespoon finely chopped red onion

1 tablespoon lime juice, 1 plum tomato

1 soft flour tortilla

salt and pepper, to taste

In separate sieves, drain the kidney beans and asparagus thoroughly. In a mixing bowl, mash the asparagus until smooth. Stir in the fromage frais, coriander, parsley, onion and lime juice. Season to taste with salt and pepper and set aside.

Quarter the tomato and scoop out the seeds. Cut the flesh into small pieces and fold into the asparagus mixture along with the kidney beans.

Lay a tortilla out on a work surface and spread with the vegetable mixture. Fold over a portion of the left hand side of the tortilla then roll up from bottom to top to give a cylinder. Eat immediately or wrap in greaseproof paper or kitchen foil and pack in a lunch box.

calories per serving: 293   fat grams per serving: 10

VEGETABLES MENESTRA

Serves 2
150g fresh or frozen peas

150g fresh or frozen broad beans

150g asparagus

1 teaspoon olive oil

1 clove garlic, chopped

25g Serrano ham, chopped

1 teaspoon flour

3 canned artichokes, halved

1 tablespoon chopped fresh parsley

To serve:
Slice of fresh rye or pumpernickel bread or a small baked potato.

Bring a large saucepan of water to the boil. Add the peas, broad beans and trimmed asparagus, return to the boil and simmer for 3 minutes until the vegetables are cooked but still quite crisp. Drain well.

Heat the oil in a large frying pan and add the chopped garlic. Cook over a medium-low heat, stirring constantly, until the garlic is just golden. Add the ham and cook, stirring, for about 3 minutes, then stir in the flour and cook for another 2–3 minutes.

Stir in the cooked vegetables, plus the artichokes and cook, stirring for another 3 minutes until the vegetables are tender and the artichokes are heated through. Transfer to a bowl and sprinkle with the chopped parsley. Serve accompanied by fresh bread or a baked potato, if desired.

calories per serving: 204   fat grams per serving: 3.5

SMOKED CHICKEN AND MEXICAN BLACK BEAN SALAD

Serves 1   150g cooked black beans

40g smoked chicken or turkey

60g red bell pepper

30g celery, any leaves reserved

15g spring onion

10g fresh coriander

1 teaspoon finely chopped green chilli

juice of 1 lime

salt and pepper, to taste

To serve:
Slice of toasted granary bread

Place the black beans in a mixing bowl. Cut the smoked chicken or turkey into strips and stir it into the beans. Finely dice the bell pepper, celery and spring onion and stir them in too.

Roughly chop the reserved celery leaves with the leaves and tender stalks of the coriander. Stir them into the salad with the green chilli. Pour in the lime juice and season to taste with salt and pepper. Transfer to a serving plate or lunch box. Serve with toasted granary bread.

calories per serving: 260   fat grams per serving: 3

SALMON PIZZA

Serves 1   75g fresh salmon fillet or 200g tin of pink salmon,

boned and skinned

1 small pizza base

1–2 tablespoons fresh tomato sauce

1 tomato

1 tablespoon chopped red onion

$1/2$ teaspoon dried red chilli flakes (optional)

3 tablespoons low-fat yoghurt

1 sprig fresh dill

Pre-heat the oven to 220°C/425°F. Trim the salmon of any skin and bones and dice the flesh. Place the pizza base on a baking tray and spread with the tomato sauce. Dice the tomato and sprinkle it over the sauce, then sprinkle with the red onion and chilli flakes. Arrange the diced salmon evenly over the top.

Bake for 15–20 minutes or until the fish is cooked and the pizza base is lightly browned. Remove from the oven, spoon on the yoghurt and garnish with fronds from the sprig of dill.

calories per serving: 365   fat grams per serving: 18

SALMON, POTATO AND ASPARAGUS SALAD

Serves 2   1 large salmon fillet

3 stalks asparagus

150g baby new potatoes

$1/2$ mango • 50g low-fat yoghurt

$1/2$ teaspoon wholegrain mustard

1 tablespoon lemon juice or white wine vinegar

1 tablespoon chopped fresh chives

$1/2$ stick celery

140g mixed salad leaves

salt and pepper, to taste

Place the salmon in a shallow pan and cover with water. Bring to the boil, then throw in the asparagus, cover and turn off the heat. Leave to stand until the cooking water reaches room temperature.

Meanwhile, in a large saucepan, place the potatoes, cover generously with water and bring to the boil. Lower the heat and simmer for 10 minutes until tender. Drain, refresh under cold running water and set aside to cool.

Chop the mango and combine in a blender with the yoghurt, mustard and lemon juice or vinegar. Process until smooth, then stir in the chives by hand. Season to taste with salt and pepper and place the dressing in the fridge to chill.

Remove the salmon and asparagus from the poaching liquid and pat dry with kitchen paper. Cut both into bite-sized pieces and place in a bowl with the cooled cooked potatoes. Chop the celery finely and add it to the bowl. Gently fold in the mango-yoghurt dressing.

Arrange the mixed salad leaves in a salad bowl, top with the dressed salmon and vegetables and serve.

calories per serving: 285   fat grams per serving: 13

PASTA WITH SPRING VEGETABLES

Serves 1   100g dried pasta such as penne

1 teaspoon vegetable bouillon powder

50g asparagus spears

50g baby carrots, or sliced regular carrots

50g baby courgettes, or sliced regular courgettes

50g mangetout or fine beans, trimmed

1 teaspoon balsamic vinegar

15g parmesan cheese, shaved

2 teaspoon basil leaves, shredded

1 teaspoon finely chopped green part of spring onion

freshly ground black pepper

Bring a large saucepan of water to the boil. Add the vegetable bouillon powder and stir to dissolve. Add the pasta and note the cooking time on the packet.

Leave the pasta to boil while you prepare the vegetables, trimming and slicing them as necessary.

Five minutes before the end of the pasta's cooking time, add the asparagus, carrots, courgettes and mangetout or beans – do not stir. Continue cooking for 5 minutes or until the pasta and vegetables are all al dente. Drain thoroughly.

Place the pasta and vegetables on a serving plate and sprinkle with the balsamic vinegar. Top with the shavings of parmesan, the basil and spring onion. Grind some black pepper over the top and serve.

calories per serving: 229   fat grams per serving: 7

HEALTHY AND HEARTY VEGETABLE STEW

Serves 4   2 teaspoons olive oil

1 onion, chopped

1/2 cabbage, chopped

2 carrots, cut into 1 inch pieces

2 celery stalks, cut into 1 inch pieces

1 courgette, cut into 1 inch pieces

4 small red potatoes (with skin), cut into 1 inch pieces

225g fresh mushrooms, sliced

6 tomatoes peeled, seeded and diced

400ml chicken stock

15g fresh chopped basil

1 tablespoon fresh thyme, chopped

salt and pepper, to taste

To serve:

1 tablespoon cottage cheese

In a large pan over a medium heat, heat the oil. Add the onion and cabbage and sauté until tender, for about 5 minutes. Add the carrots, celery, courgette, potatoes and mushrooms and simmer for 5 minutes. Add the tomatoes, stock, basil, thyme and salt and pepper, to taste. Bring to the boil, then reduce the heat to low and simmer until the potatoes are tender, for about 20–30 minutes.

Pour the soup into serving bowls and add the cottage cheese on top.

Note: Alternatively you can serve the soup with a small grilled, poached or roast chicken breast, or ½ cup of cooked butter beans or chick peas or 100 grams of cubed tofu. This will ensure you get a good balance of starch and protein.

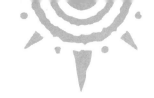

CHAPTER TEN

Body Blitz 14-Day Eating Plan

Now that you have read all about the Body Blitz diet, this chapter will show you how to start putting the diet into practice. I have designed the 14-day eating plan for you to see day by day how you can apply the nutritional strategies that we have discussed throughout the book. Here is a quick recap of the strategies:

- **Operate the starch curfew** – no bread, pasta, rice, potatoes or cereal after 5 p.m.
- **Decrease overall fat intake** – aim for no more than 40 grams of fat a day.
- **Eat your fruit and vegetables** – aim for five portions of fruit and vegetables a day.
- **Reduce the amount of calories you consume** – aim for a daily calorie intake of between 1200–1500 calories.
- **Drink two litres of water** – spread evenly throughout the day.

Daily Calorie Allowance

The Body Blitz daily calorie allowance is between 1200–1500 calories. Here is how the calorie allowance breaks down for each meal:

breakfast: 300–350 calories
lunch: 350–400 calories
dinner: 500–550 calories

snacks: 150–200 calories (if you have a smoothie as a snack your calorie intake will be higher. Don't worry about this – as we discussed in Step Five the **80–20 rule** gives you a 500 calorie cushion each day).

These are only guidelines and you don't need to stick to them rigidly. Remember, the Body Blitz diet contains strategies which give you the flexibility to fit the diet into your lifestyle, whilst still achieving *your* weight loss goals.

BODY BLITZ BREAKFASTS

As we saw in Step One it is important to start your day with a healthy breakfast. Here are some further suggestions for delicious Body Blitz breakfasts. Each breakfast contains less than 350 calories.

piece of fruit; slice of pumpernickel bread; 100g low-fat cottage cheese
ginseng tea followed by a fruit smoothie (see opposite)
1 English muffin, split and toasted, spread thinly with quark and topped with a sliced plum
1 slice of wholemeal toast grilled with 25g Edam cheese and sliced tomato; small glass of orange juice.
2 grilled tomatoes with 2 rashers grilled bacon with fat cut off; 1 slice of wholemeal toast
1 'skinny' American muffin with skimmed milk cappuccino

BODY BLITZ BREAKFAST SMOOTHIES

As we have already seen smoothies play an important role in the Body Blitz diet. Not only are they great as a mid-afternoon snack but they also make a delicious, filling and portable breakfast. Why not invest in a thermos flask or travelling mug so you can enjoy your smoothie when you are on the move!

Smoothies are very quick and easy to make – just follow these steps:

1. Open a small tin of fruit in natural juice and pour contents into a blender.

2. Add a handful of your favourite breakfast cereal, for example, bran flakes, oatmeal, muesli, Special K or add $1/2$ tablespoon of wheatgerm.

3. Add 100g of plain or fruit low-fat yoghurt.

4. Add 200 ml skimmed milk, or unsweetened soya milk or skimmed goats milk.

5. Blend and go!

Top Tip

Making your smoothie with frozen fruit will give it an extra creamy smoothness and thickness. Freeze the tinned fruit on a tray – remember to separate the fruit first to make it easier to handle when frozen. Similarly, you can freeze the juice of the fruit and/or the low-fat yoghurt in an ice cube tray and add the frozen cubes to your smoothie.

Here are some delicious fruit and cereal combos for your breakfast smoothies:

- banana with oatmeal
- apricots with malted flakes, for example, Special K
- peaches with shreddies
- prunes with bran flakes
- raspberries with wheatgerm

BODY BLITZ LUNCHES

As we discussed in Step One it is really important to eat some protein in your midday meal, ideally in a ratio of one portion of starch to one portion of protein. This improves your concentration, fuels you with energy for the afternoon and helps you avoid those mid-afternoon sugar cravings. The suggestions in Step One as well as the recipes in the *Eating In* chapter contain a wide range of ideas for your midday meal. Here are some further tips and suggestions.

SANDWICHES

Sandwiches are great to have at lunchtime. Open sandwiches are better than the traditional closed sandwiches as they give an excellent balance of starch and protein as well as containing fewer calories. Here are some suggestions for delicious open sandwiches – each sandwich contains less than 350 calories. To ensure you get your quota of vegetables you can pile up on the vegetable sandwich filling or munch with a cup of vegetable crudités.

Note: See page 53 for how much a portion of starch and protein is. As we discussed earlier, you can also visually estimate portion sizes – a portion of starch looks roughly the same size as a portion of protein. This means with open sandwiches you need to add a layer of protein, such as tuna, chicken or tinned salmon, approximately the same thickness as the slice of bread or the roll.

Select one of the following:	Pile on:	Add a portion of one of the following:
• small pitta bread • medium granary roll split in two • small bagel, toasted • thin slice of wholemeal bread • small slice of focaccia bread	lettuce chopped tomatoes diced peppers grated carrots chopped spring onions cucumber slices alfalfa sprouts beansprouts	• tinned tuna in brine • poached egg • chargrilled chicken breast • flavoured cottage cheese • smoked salmon • tinned pink salmon • tinned pilchards in tomato sauce • lean sliced smoked ham • peeled boiled prawns • grated Edam cheese

As you cut down on the amount of fat you are consuming in the form of butter, margarine spreads and mayonnaise, you may feel that your sandwiches are dry and lacking in taste. Here are some low-fat spreads that will help keep your sandwiches moist and tasty!

marmite
thin scraping of quark
fromage frais mixed with tomato salsa
natural yoghurt mixed with a little balsamic vinegar
grainy mustard
reduced fat tsatziki
tomato salsa
fromage frais or low-fat natural yoghurt mixed with teaspoon of sweet Thai chilli sauce
mango chutney

But remember, the Body Blitz diet is not about cutting all fat from your diet – the essential fats are important and you can get these in sandwich toppings such as salmon and tinned pilchards – and of course you can have a small amount of olive oil dressing on a side salad.

AND DON'T FORGET ABOUT SOUPS

Soups can make a nourishing and filling meal at any time of the year, but as the weather gets colder soups can be a particularly satisfying, quick and portable meal. And with the extensive range of pre-prepared fresh soups (found at the chill cabinet of your supermarket) and tinned soups available you really can be spoilt for choice.

Select vegetable and broth-based soups with less than 300 calories per serving or make your own hearty vegetable stew (see recipe on page 214). Avoid cream-based soups and always read the food labels. If you have not already got one, invest in a thermos flask so you can enjoy your soup wherever you go.

Beans or tofu are delicious added to soups and both are great sources of protein. If you are eating soup at lunchtime, serve with a portion of starch, for example, a slice of wholemeal, rye or soda bread.

STARCH CURFEW DINNERS

As we discussed in Step One the basic principle behind your **starch curfew** dinner is to omit the starches and eat instead protein (lean meat, poultry, fish, eggs and pulses) with vegetables and fruit. The recipes in the *Eating In* chapter contain some interesting ideas, which you can use as treats or when having friends for supper. Or you can put the starch curfew into practice by simply following these guidelines:

Select one protein food from the following list:

- 150g lean meat, all visible fat cut off, or poultry
- 150g white fish or shellfish, for example, cod, peeled prawns, plaice

- 100g oily fish, for example, mackerel, salmon, tuna, herring, pilchards
- 2 eggs
- 150g cooked pulses, for example, kidney beans, lentils, chick peas, haricot beans

Avoid: high fat content meats such as sausages and trim fat off meat before cooking.

Serve with unlimited vegetables: The list below will give you some ideas:
Cabbage, carrots, peas, cauliflower, lettuce, spinach, tomatoes, watercress, fennel, courgettes, leeks, brussels sprouts, broccoli, runner beans, beansprouts, water chestnuts, sweet corn, mushrooms, broad beans, onions, peppers, marrow, pumpkin, turnip, to name just a few.

Select one of the following cooking methods:

| braise | steam | bake | microwave | boil |
| dry roast | casserole | grill | poach | |

Avoid frying and watch out for stir-frying and sautéing as this can add an enormous amount of fat and calories. Do not add additional fat or oils to vegetables.

Sweet Tooth?: Finish your meal with fresh fruit, a low-fat yoghurt or fruit sorbet.

Daily Allowance

Each day you must have:

Half a pint of skimmed or semi-skimmed milk or 150g pot of low-fat yoghurt
No more than two cups of tea or coffee a day
Two litres of water spread evenly throughout the day
Five portions of fruit and vegetables.

14-DAY EATING PLAN

	Breakfast	**Lunch**	**Dinner**	**Optional Snacks**
Day 1	porridge made with 1 teacup of porridge oats and 1 teacup of milk; serve with 1 chopped apple small glass of freshly squeezed orange juice	smoked chicken and Mexican black bean salad *(see recipe on page 211)*; serve with slice of toasted granary bread slice of melon	* starch curfew main course; serve with salad or vegetables of your choice small bowl of fruit sorbet	can of tomato juice 150g pot of low-fat fruit yoghurt
Day 2	1 teacup of Special K with skimmed milk from allowance and handful of raspberries small glass of orange juice	any carton of fresh vegetable soup under 300 calories; add $1/2$ cup of kidney beans and serve with 2 crispbreads 1 pear	* starch curfew main course; serve with salad or vegetables of your choice small bowl of stewed fruit	1 apple 150g pot of low-fat fruit yoghurt
Day 3	$1/2$ grapefruit with teaspoon of sugar porridge made with milk (same as day 1)	open sandwich with meat, fish or cheese (under 350 calories); serve with small bag of vegetable crudités with salsa 1 apple	* starch curfew main course; serve with salad or vegetables of your choice slice of pineapple	small glass orange juice 1 kiwi fruit

	Breakfast	Lunch	Dinner	Optional Snacks
Day 4	large bowl of fresh fruit salad 1 slice of wholemeal toast spread with a thin layer of quark and reduced sugar jam	medium size jacket potato topped with small pot of low-fat cottage cheese; serve with small green salad small glass of orange or apple juice	* starch curfew main course; serve with salad or vegetables of your choice small bowl of stewed fruit	banana smoothie 1 apple
Day 5	porridge made with water; add a handful chopped apple; serve with 2 tablespoons of natural yoghurt	open sandwich with meat, fish or cheese (under 350 calories) small glass of orange juice or apple juice	* starch curfew main course; serve with salad or vegetables of your choice small bowl of fruit sorbet	1 kiwi fruit 1 pear
Day 6	1/2 grapefruit with 1/2 teaspoon of sugar 1 slice wholemeal toast with marmite and cottage cheese	large bowl of hearty vegetable stew (see recipe on page 214) 150g pot of low-fat fruit yoghurt	* starch curfew main course; serve with salad or vegetables of your choice 1 banana	can of vegetable juice 1 orange

	Breakfast	**Lunch**	**Dinner**	**Optional Snacks**
Day 7	large bowl of fresh fruit salad 2 Ryvita with thin scraping of quark and topped with sliced plum	poached egg with 1 toasted bagel small glass of orange or apple juice	* starch curfew main course; serve with salad or vegetables of your choice small bowl of fruit sorbet	150g pot natural bio yoghurt with 1 teaspoon of honey 1 kiwi fruit
Day 8	porridge made with water; serve with 2 table-spoons of natural bio yoghurt and 1 chopped apple small glass freshly squeezed orange juice	mixed medium sushi box (250g) small glass of orange or apple juice	* starch curfew main course; serve with salad or vegetables of your choice 150g pot of low-fat fruit fromage frais	cup of grapes 1 can of vegetable juice
Day 9	large bowl of fresh fruit salad with 150g pot low-fat bio yoghurt	Mexican-style wraps with beans, herbs and vegetables (see recipe on page 209) low-fat chocolate mousse	* starch curfew main course; serve with salad or vegetables of your choice small bowl of fruit sorbet	300ml shop bought fruit smoothie 1 banana

	Breakfast	**Lunch**	**Dinner**	**Optional Snacks**
Day 10	swiss muesli made with ½ cup of porridge oats soaked overnight with milk from allowance and 1 teacup of water, mixed with small handful of sultanas, a grated apple and a pinch of nutmeg	homemade chef salad made wtih 28g lean chicken breast, 28g lean ham, 56g cottage cheese, lettuce, tomatoes, onion, cucumbers and peppers; serve with 1 slice of rye bread 1 pear	* starch curfew main course; serve with salad or vegetables of your choice small bowl of stewed fruit	1 kiwi fruit 1 can of vegetable juice
Day 11	1 cup of bran flakes cereal with skimmed milk from allowance and small banana	1 medium jacket potato with 150g pot cottage cheese with chopped tomato and fresh basil leaves; serve with a side salad or bag of vegetable sticks small glass of orange or apple juice	* starch curfew main course; serve with salad or vegetables of your choice slice of melon	1 cup of seedless grapes 150g pot of low-fat bio yoghurt

	Breakfast	Lunch	Dinner	Optional Snacks
Day 12	swiss muesli with sultanas and grated apple (same as Day 10)	1 slice wholemeal toast with small tin of baked beans and 2 grilled tomatoes small glass of orange or apple juice	* starch curfew main course; serve with salad or vegetables of your choice small bowl of pineapple in natural juice	150g pot of low-fat bio yoghurt slice of melon
Day 13	large fresh fruit salad with 150g pot natural low-fat bio yoghurt	toasted bagel with 2 slices smoked trout or salmon; serve with green salad slice of melon	* starch curfew main course; serve with salad or vegetables of your choice low-fat chocolate mousse	1 small banana small glass of orange or apple juice
Day 14	1 poached egg on 1 slice dry wholemeal toast small glass of orange juice	medium size jacket potato with small can of tuna in brine and small green salad 1 pear	* starch curfew main course; serve with salad or vegetables of your choice small bowl of fruit sorbet	1 apple 150g pot of low-fat bio yoghurt

* Choose any of the **starch curfew** dinner recipes from the *Eating In* chapter or create your own main course using the starch curfew guidelines discussed earlier.

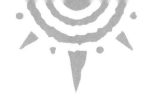

Useful Addresses

Activeaction.com,
PO Box 32926,
London, SW20 8FS
E-mail: queries@activeaction.com
Website: www.activeaction.com
Joanna Hall's web site providing active assistance software, products and courses to help individuals achieve healthier lifestyle goals.

Tanita Uk Ltd,
The Barn, Philpots Close,
Yiewsley, West Drayton,
Middlesex, UB7 7RY
Tel: 0800 7316994
Manufacturers of Tanita Body fat monitors. Available to purchase from larger Boots stores, John Lewis, Argos, Alders, Innovations and fitness stores.

British Heart Foundation,
National Centre for Physical Activity
and Health,
Loughborough University of Technology,
Loughborough, LE11 3TU
Tel: 01509 223259
E-mail: l.almond@lboro.ac.uk
A telephone helpline will be available in 2001 to provide information on incorporating greater physical activity levels into every day lifestyles.

Sport England,
16 Upper Woburn Place,
London, WC1H OQP
Provides programmes and initiatives to incorporate greater involvement in exercise and sport.

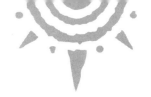

Index